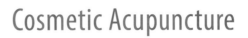

Cosmetic Acupuncture

of related interest

Facial Enhancement Acupuncture
Clinical Use and Application
Paul Adkins
ISBN 978 1 84819 129 7
eISBN 978 0 85701 103 9

Japanese Holistic Face Massage
Rosemary Patten
ISBN 978 1 84819 122 8
eISBN 978 0 85701 100 8

Vital Face
Facial Exercises and Massage for Health and Beauty
Leena Kiviluoma
ISBN 978 1 84819 166 2
eISBN 978 0 85701 130 5

Acupuncture and Chinese Medicine
Roots of Modern Practice
Charles Buck
ISBN 978 1 84819 159 4
eISBN 978 0 85701 133 6

The Active Points Test
A Clinical Test for Identifying and Selecting Effective
Points for Acupuncture and Related Therapies
Stefano Marcelli
ISBN 978 1 84819 233 1
eISBN 978 0 85701 207 4

The Handbook of Five Element Practice
Nora Franglen
ISBN 978 1 84819 188 4
eISBN 978 0 85701 145 9

Needling Techniques for Acupuncturists
Basic Principles and Techniques
Edited by Xiaorong Chang
ISBN 978 1 84819 057 3
eISBN 978 0 85701 045 2

Cosmetic Acupuncture

A Traditional Chinese Medicine Approach to
Cosmetic and Dermatological Problems

SECOND EDITION

Radha Thambirajah

SINGING
DRAGON

LONDON AND PHILADELPHIA

First published in 2016
by Jessica Kingsley Publishers
73 Collier Street
London N1 9BE, UK
and
400 Market Street, Suite 400
Philadelphia, PA 19106, USA

www.jkp.com

Disclaimer: Every effort has been made to ensure that the information contained in this book is correct, but it should not in any way be substituted for medical advice. Readers should always consult a qualified medical practitioner before adopting any complementary or alternative therapies. Neither the author nor the publisher takes responsibility for any consequences of any decision made as a result of the information contained in this book.

Library of Congress Cataloging in Publication Data
Thambirajah, Radha, author.
  Cosmetic acupuncture : a traditional Chinese medicine approach to cosmetic and dermatological problems / Radha Thambirajah. -- Second edition.
       p. ; cm.
  Includes bibliographical references and index.
  ISBN 978-1-84819-267-6 (alk. paper)
  I. Title.
  [DNLM: 1. Acupuncture Therapy. 2. Cosmetic Techniques. 3. Medicine, Chinese Traditional. 4. Skin Diseases--therapy. WB 369]
  RL87
  615.8'92--dc23
                            2015010864

British Library Cataloguing in Publication Data
A CIP catalogue record for this book is available from the British Library

ISBN 978 1 84819 267 6
eISBN 978 0 85701 215 9

Printed and bound in China

To my loving son,
SATHYAN

CONTENTS

ABOUT THE AUTHOR

Radha Thambirajah graduated from Shanghai Medical College in 1970, where she studied medicine and specialized in acupuncture. Following her internship in China, she returned to Sri Lanka and pioneered the practice of acupuncture. In 1980 she founded the Academy of Chinese Acupuncture in Sri Lanka. She has been teaching and training doctors and health professionals all over the world for over 30 years.

In 1984, she moved to England and continued her teaching and clinical work. For the past 25 years, she has lectured in Germany, Spain, Switzerland, Italy, Denmark and Norway for a number of teaching organizations, universities and acupuncture societies.

Her first book, *Energetics in Acupuncture*, was published in German in 2005, and has been translated into Spanish.

Radha practises in Sutton Coldfield, West Midlands, UK.

PREFACE

It is not possible to separate the issue of beauty from skin and connective tissue problems and issues concerning general health. In fact, it was by accident that I realized, back in the 1970s, that acupuncture is effective not only for the treatment of general diseases but also for improving general appearance.

At that time, I was offering free treatment to patients in Sri Lanka who could not afford to pay. Patients with chronic diseases such as arthritis, bronchial asthma and skin problems came frequently for acupuncture, sometimes even four or five times a week. I noticed that after two or three weeks of regular treatment patients often looked different – there was a spring in their step and their eyes shone; in fact, they looked more beautiful, more cheerful and less strained.

It was at about the same time that I began using acupuncture to treat cosmetic problems such as improving muscle tone after childbirth or after losing weight. The results were extremely good, but did not last long. It slowly dawned on me that, to maintain the results, patients needed to change their diet and do a little bit of homework. Furthermore, acupuncture at some points on the body was required to balance their energy. A combination of working from within and from outside gave the best and most lasting results.

When I came to the West, I faced greater challenges. Patients wanted to look perfect – and therefore we had more imperfections to work on. I began to understand the inter-relationship between the skin and the connective tissue; the difference between fatty skin and moist skin; how there could be a mixture of dry skin in one part of the body but oily skin in another part; how one could treat cellulite in a slim person. Patients with eczema, psoriasis and acne were common in my practice, and I perfected my skills on them. As my practice in England was private, I had fewer patients to treat than I had in Sri Lanka – and therefore more time for each patient. I took time to advise on diet and carry out extensive energy-balancing treatment with acupuncture. The results were rewarding, and once, after having cured a 71-year-old woman who had suffered all her life with neurodermatitis, I believed that I was ready to share my experiences with other therapists.

What I have learned through my experiences is that cosmetic acupuncture is not about beauty but about health. If our interior is healthy and balanced, and if we have inner tranquillity and contentment, if we are well nourished and exercise moderately, our inner beauty will shine through.

Every part of our body needs good blood circulation, moisture, free movement of fluid and the ability to eliminate secretions, and no stagnation of dampness (which results in a puffy appearance). The skin, however, which is the outermost covering of our body, is visible in a very large area, and therefore is the most important place to manifest beauty. When treating skin problems, one must take into account the various internal organs that influence it. An imbalance in the energy system of internal organs may result in a skin disease or a flawed appearance. When this imbalance is corrected, the skin disease or the flaw disappears.

This means that good results can be obtained by treating not the local area affected by a skin disease or imperfection, but the energy imbalance that causes the problem. Thus, local needles are not necessary to treat acne vulgaris. Rather, the treatment of acne involves the application of needles to points on other parts of the body to reduce oiliness and the inflammation of facial skin. This, combined with avoidance of foods that cause oily skin and increased consumption of foods to regulate bowel movements (as this also helps the skin to eliminate its sebaceous secretions), results in successful long-term effects. But, of course, if local needles around the area of the acne are used at the same time, the results will also be instantaneous. Patients want to see immediate results (especially in cosmetic therapy) but they also want long-term effectiveness.

Therefore, it becomes important to bring about a state of balance to the body, but also to have the 'know-how' to treat the cosmetic and dermatological problems locally in order to cure them. I hope to do exactly this. In the first half of this book, I explain the blood, energy and body fluid states of all the internal organs relevant to cosmetic therapy and the treatment of dermatological conditions; in the second half, I deal with common skin problems and cosmetic problems and describe local therapies for these.

Radha Thambirajah

THE 12 ORGANS (ZANG FU) AND THEIR ABBREVIATIONS

GB	Gall Bladder	LI	Large Intestine
P	Pericardium	St	Stomach
H	Heart	Liv	Liver
SI	Small Intestine	TW	Triple Warmer
K	Kidney	Lu	Lung
Sp	Spleen	UB	Urinary Bladder

CHAPTER 1

THE BLOOD, YIN, YANG AND QI IN ALL ORGANS

CHAPTER CONTENTS

1.1 YIN AND YANG

The yin and yang are the two sides – or duality – in every object, person or natural phenomenon. Everything around us can be described as yin or yang in nature. These two sides exist together, always, albeit in different proportions – thus, it is safe to say that something is yin dominant or yang dominant in nature. However, we cannot say that something is purely yin or yang in nature because the yin and yang are always found together, and if one is not present the other will lose the condition for its existence.

The yin and yang exist together, and are related to each other, causing changes when one aspect grows or the other diminishes. These states are described as yin or yang dominant, yin excess or yang deficiency, and so on. The dominance of one gives the yin or yang character to an object or phenomenon.

If we can understand this relationship, we can predict the possible changes. In traditional Chinese medicine, sickness is described as an imbalance between yin and yang. The imbalance can be brought back to balance by acupuncture, diet, change in lifestyle or use of herbal medicine.

In this book we talk about yin and yang in detail, and also about Blood and Qi, in order to understand different dermatological and cosmetic problems and their solutions.

Yin and yang in balance

TABLE 1.1 COMPONENTS OF YIN AND YANG

Yin	Yang
Cold	Hot
Passive	Active
Damp	Dry
Solid	Hollow
Ascending	Descending
Contracting	Dispersing
Nutrition	Protection
Substance	Function

I will now examine each of the characteristics featured in Table 1.1.

1.1.1 Yin

Cold

Generally speaking, this means that the patient feels cold or feels cold to the therapist's touch but it also refers to symptoms that worsen during cold weather or on exposure to cold (e.g. when the air conditioning is activated on a warm day). Cold causes the skin to adopt a pale or blue appearance; if inflammation such as tendonitis or cellulitis is present, then the skin may exhibit pale, blue and reddish marbling.

Cold is generally caused by yang deficiency or by Blood deficiency, i.e. there is insufficient Blood to circulate warmth around the body.

Passive

This refers to an inactive person or a hypoactive organ, or a symptom that worsens during rest or passivity.

Moderate exercise and physical activity warm the body, bringing colour to the cheeks and moisture to the skin through sweating. They also improve the metabolism and function of the heart and other internal organs. They firm the muscles and improve the functional energy (Qi). Lack of exercise has the opposite effect – the circulation of blood and fluid is sluggish and does not reach the periphery, the skin appears pale and dull, and organs are slow in function. Skin symptoms of a yin-dominant nature tend to stay fixed in one or two sites and change little over a long period.

Wet

This refers to *thin fluid* that moistens the skin surface, the mucous membranes and the tendons, giving them softness and elasticity. An excess of wetness could be caused by water retention, or hyperhidrosis (see page 155), or can be the result of poor skin function – leading to open pores even when it is not warm.

This term also refers to stagnation of *thick fluid*, such as sebaceous secretions, oedema and cellulite, or fat tissue under the skin. Another term for this thick fluid is phlegm. The thick or the fatty fluids may result from excessive consumption of oily foods or refined sugar and carbohydrates.

Solid

This is a term that describes the yin internal organs, but it can also be used to describe the appearance of cysts and tumours that result from stagnation of thick fluids. These solid forms result from two causes:

- The functional energy (Qi) becomes retarded because of a diet high in cold and raw foods that slows down metabolism, and because of excessive fatty foods and milk products combined with no exercise. This causes stagnation and excessive thick fluids, which form into solid tumours and cysts.

- The thin fluids within the thick fluids dry out, causing them to become too thick, too solid, with resulting difficulty in flowing.

Descending

Cold and wet have a downward movement. If one warms a pot of water on a fire, the warm water moves upwards while the water at the bottom of the pot, although it is closer to the heat source, is colder. Oedema, for example, acts in the same way, manifesting more often in the lower extremities.

Skin diseases restricted to the lower parts of the body, in contrast to those occurring in the upper parts, are more commonly yin diseases (e.g. eczema, fungal infections in the perineum, varicose eczema and ulcers). The separating point between the upper and lower body is considered to be the navel. Typically, arthritic joint pains of a yin-dominant nature also manifest in the lower joints rather than in the neck and arms.

Contracting

Cold causes us to curl up into the foetal position. Thus, illnesses such as Parkinson's disease, ankylosing spondylitis, osteoporosis and depression, which cause patients to assume this particular posture, are said to be yin diseases.

However, 'contracting' also refers to the fact that skin closes and muscles tighten when cold, and energy moves towards the interior, leaving the exterior without sufficient Blood or warmth. This means that the immune system (the Wei Qi), which should be at the skin surface to protect the body from external climatic pathogenic factors, becomes less powerful.

Nutrition

The Spleen and the Stomach are the most important nourishing organs of the body, and they nourish all organs and tissues of the body. The Spleen stores the nutrition from the food and drink we consume, and distributes this nutrition through the blood to all parts of the body, particularly the periphery. Thus, conditions such as thin and wrinkly skin or dry and cracked lips or heels can have one of two causes: (1) inadequate nutrition, i.e. a lack of protein, milk products or carbohydrate in the diet; or (2) poor distribution of nutrition – poor functional Qi of the Spleen – due to a diet of cold and raw food, or eating too much too late in the evenings.

Again, faulty nutrition, such as excessive consumption of refined carbohydrates and sugar, or of fatty and oily foods, can result in a fatty and thick skin, giving the appearance of unclean skin and affecting the function of the sebaceous glands and their secretions to the skin surface.

Substance

This refers to fluid, nutrition, Blood or waste matter that is either in constant circulation or is part of the elimination cycle. This term also can relate to body weight, quantity of stool, urine and menstrual bleeding. The more substance there is, the more yin there is, and vice versa.

1.1.2 Yang

Hot

This means that the diseased area is hot to the touch and red in colour or the patient feels hot or burning.

In skin diseases, for example, eczema, acne and urticaria, heat can be caused by inflammation or allergies.

Heat symptoms can also be caused by a state of yin deficiency, when the yang is relatively dominant and occasionally increases even further because of poor control. In this case, dryness would also be present.

Active

A normal amount of activity in an organ or a person would not be an imbalanced state, but being *hyperactive* is a yang-dominant symptom. Hyperactivity can be caused by a simple yang excess state or by a yin deficiency state, causing recurrent episodes of rising, uncontrolled yang.

This would result in the skin being hypersensitive and reacting quickly to allergens. Sweating, for example, could be quick and excessive when hot.

Yang-dominant symptoms tend to travel over the body (wandering nature), whereas yin symptoms remain confined to one area.

We should be concerned not just about the black and white areas (i.e. either extremely slow or fast activity) but also about the grey areas (i.e. small changes) as these also represent problems. In Western medicine, doctors strive to lower blood cholesterol levels to below 4 mmol/L but do not consider a pulse rate of 85 or passing stools only twice a week to be a problem. In traditional Chinese medicine, it is important to detect and treat *tendencies* towards yin- or yang-dominant states, because these are easier to cure. A very severe imbalance or one that has been treated aggressively with medication is very difficult to cure.

Dry

This means that there is less thin fluid, so a yin deficiency (thus a yang dominance). Symptoms include dry or hard skin with peeling or cracks, and sparse, straw-like body hair.

Dry skin looks old and ages fast, and many thin wrinkles appear in these affected areas. The skin around the eyes, mouth, elbows, knees, hands and feet is especially prone to dryness. People who spend time in the sun tend to have dry skin on the exposed areas of their body.

Hollow

This again refers to the yang internal organs, which are mainly functional organs such as the intestines and the bladder. Skin that is not firm and can be pinched upwards like tissue paper is caused by a nutritional deficiency.

Ascending

Heat has an upwards disposition. Dryness causes lightness, which will also rise. Therefore, yang-dominant symptoms tend to manifest primarily in the upper part of the body. Examples include eczema or neurodermatitis on the face, neck, thorax and arms, and also urticaria and acne. Interestingly, the skin in the lower part of the body is often quite clear, the level of the navel being the point of division between the upper and lower body.

Dispersing

Sweating is perhaps the best example of a dispersing function. Dispersion involves moving from the interior to the exterior; a food allergy that manifests as urticaria would be a good example – even though the pathogenic factor is consumed internally, the body reaction is manifested externally.

Dispersion is a healthy reaction of the immune system, which eliminates disease-causing factors. Excess heat or fever can be eliminated by skin function.

When dispersion is not good, pathogenic factors stay in the interior and cause injury to the skin and internal organs.

Protection

The skin is our armour and protects the body from attack by external factors. As the skin is directly associated with the Lung, a poor immune system – a poor Wei Qi – means poor Lung function. However, this can be strengthened by tonifying (increasing) the yang of the Lung.

Function

Function is what we call Qi. Function and substance go together. For example, if blood is the substance, then circulation would be the function; if water is the substance, then its distribution and elimination is the function. If there is excess fluid in the body, urination should increase; when there is dryness in the body, urination should reduce – this demonstrates good function of the Kidneys.

Consider the earlier example of sweating: it is possible for someone to sweat spontaneously, especially in the cold areas of the body, thus making these areas colder. This is caused by poor function, as opening the skin to eliminate sweat and closing the skin to stop sweating are both functions of the skin. Good function is for it to be able to decide correctly when it should disperse and when it should not.

The yin and yang relate constantly and predictably to each other, creating continuous changes in the energy state. These changes are called contradiction, inter-consumption, lack of control and consequent hyperactivity of yang or stagnation of yin, and inter-transformation. These relationships are covered in detail in my previous book, *Energetics of Acupuncture.*

It is important to appreciate the different ways in which the yin and yang relate to each other, otherwise it will be very difficult to understand the rest of this book.

1.2 BLOOD, YIN, YANG AND QI

Having briefly encountered the yin and yang, we now need to consider them in more detail. We can diagramatically represent yin and yang by two 'towers', providing an easy visualization of an imbalanced state. We can also split the yin and yang towers into two extra columns, called *Blood* and *Qi,* and we will work with these four towers throughout this book, which will increase our understanding and application of therapy points. We will be able to see clearly the imbalance we are working with, and the required therapy – what needs to be tonified or sedated – will become clear as we analyze these towers.

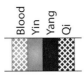

The terms Blood, yin, yang and Qi are used in many books and by numerous practitioners. However, each person who reads these terms will understand them in their own unique way. Therefore, I wish to explain in advance what I personally mean by these four terms (Table 1.2), so that it will be clear to the reader.

TABLE 1.2 BLOOD, YIN, YANG AND QI

Blood	Yin	Yang	Qi
Nutrition	Moisture	Heat	Function
Skin thickness	Skin moisture	Skin temperature	Opening and closing function of pores
Thick fluid	Thin fluid	Inflammation	Adaptation to temperature changes
Sebaceous secretion	Sweat fluidity	Redness	Firming, holding in
Vulnerability	Dryness	Paleness	Sensitivity
Healing	Cracking, peeling	Marbling	Elimination when necessary

Now, let us consider each of these one by one.

1.2.1 Blood

The term Blood refers to red blood, which nourishes all the cells of the body. This red blood is *nourished by the Spleen*, which stores the nutrition from food and drink and distributes it to the whole body; it is *synthesized by the Heart*, which combines the nutrition with fluid and oxygen and circulates it; and it is *stored in the Blood vessels and released by the Liver* when any part of the body needs Blood, or if there is any bleeding.

Blood is nourished from food and drink by the Spleen and from air by the Lungs.

The Kidneys make bone marrow, which makes Blood, but this Blood is not oxygenated, and therefore not called red blood.

Blood is synthesized by Heart Qi, which combines the different nutrients to make red (oxygenated) blood: this is called Heart Blood.

Blood is circulated centrally by Heart Qi and peripherally by Spleen Qi.

The Liver yin stores Blood within itself and within the vessels, and the Liver yang and Qi releases it out of the vessels (for the body to have energy) and out of the body (when bleeding). The Blood within the Liver and the vessels is called Liver Blood.

But the term Blood also stands for *nutrition*, without which any organ or tissue cannot continue to function, and would soon become exhausted. For example, osteoporosis would be a nutritional deficiency of the bones, which in terms of traditional Chinese medicine means the Kidneys have a Blood deficiency (as Kidneys nourish the bones). The skin is nourished by Blood from the Lungs (and the Lungs receive nutrition from the mother organ, the Spleen). If the Blood in the Lungs (and in the Spleen) is deficient, then the skin will become pale, thin, easy to break and slow to heal, and will be vulnerable to injuries and weather exposure.

The term Blood also means nutrition.

Heart Blood nourishes the blood vessels, the mind and its function, the tongue and speech. Heart Blood deficiency causes paleness, coldness, endogenous depression, poor concentration and memory and restless sleep.

Lung Blood nourishes the skin and body hair, and the respiratory organs. Lung Blood deficiency causes thin, vulnerable skin with less body hair, breathlessness and low energy.

Spleen Blood nourishes the entire body (mostly the muscles and fat), the lips, the extremities and the digestive system. Spleen Blood deficiency results in a person being thin or undernourished and having problems absorbing nutrition.

Kidney Blood nourishes the bones and cartilage, the head hair, the brain and nervous system and the urinary system. In people with Kidney Blood deficiency, the bones fracture easily and heal poorly, and such individuals also suffer from hair loss or thin hair, low vitality and poorly formed eggs or sperm.

Liver Blood nourishes the tendons and the eyes and fuels the function of muscle movement and stress. Liver Blood is lost during bleeding and can stagnate in the vessels (especially veins) when there is a mechanical obstruction in the circulation, or when circulation (Liver Qi) is sluggish. Blood deficiency causes paleness, tiredness, contracture and easy rupture of tendons, blurred vision and scanty menstruation with long menstrual cycles.

Symptoms of Blood deficiency are paleness, coldness, long menstrual cycles with scanty bleeding in women, poor endurance in physical and mental functions, and numbness of the extremities during rest, improving with movement. Patients are quickly exhausted and wound healing is poor.

Blood deficiency could start off different reactions in the yin, yang and Qi of the organ. To show some examples:

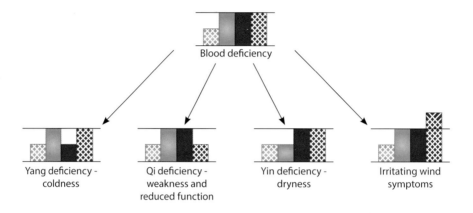

Blood deficiency can cause yang deficiency

As Blood circulates nutrition and warmth to the body, when there is less Blood coldness can result. The coldness is generalized, but manifests more in the upper body and hands. It should be stressed that it is an inner coldness associated with paleness, mental fatigue, poor concentration and memory, anxiety and depression. There could also be dizziness and some fainting.

The most common symptom of a yang deficiency is coldness.

Blood deficiency can cause Qi (function) deficiency

Blood nourishes and fuels all organs and tissues, and continues to fuel their function (Qi). Heart Blood fuels the function of concentration, intelligence, speech and mental activity. When there is a Blood deficiency, any mental work seems too much to cope with.

The function (Qi) of the Heart is to synthesize and circulate Blood. When Blood becomes deficient, the functions of Blood-building and circulation slow down, and the Heart undergoes great strain to supply the body with its nutritional needs. There can be tachyarrhythmia when stressed.

Patients have difficulty concentrating or speaking for long periods of time, and tire quickly. They constantly feel sleepy – a situation which does not improve with more sleep.

LUNG QI DEFICIENCY

Lung Blood deficiency will mean that the skin is thin and poorly nourished, and this will reduce the Lung functional Qi.

The Lung Qi controls the opening and closing functions of the skin pores, thus aiding adaptation to change in climatic temperature and maintaining a good immune system. There could also be spontaneous sweating, whether the person is cold or hot, because the skin has lost the ability to regulate the function of its pores.

Blood deficiency can cause yin deficiency

A large part of Blood is fluid. Because of this, and the fact that nutrition is now low, Blood deficiency can cause dryness, especially in the skin, hair and nails.

As this dryness is caused by Blood deficiency, it cannot be improved by increasing intake of water – only by improving Blood.

In skin problems such as neurodermatitis and generalized idiopathic itching, this type of dryness is very common.

Faulty nutrition – such as excess consumption of fatty foods, milk products and refined sugars and carbohydrates – make the skin oily and thick, and there is difficulty eliminating sebaceous secretion and sweat through the thickness, thus reducing the Qi (function) of the skin and creating the possibility of dampness and heat. If thick fluid does not circulate but stands still, this could cause damp-heat symptoms such as acne pustules or infected eczema.

Though dampness and Blood are not the same, blood is also a thick fluid. Therefore, the same rules for circulation and thinning apply to both. Both can be thinned out by consuming more water or thin fluids (and tonifying the yin by using the Front-Mu point and the Luo-connecting point of the yin organ of the element), and both can be circulated with points such as St 40, Back-Shu point or the Luo-connecting point of the yang organ of the associated element (see Glossary for an explanation of these points).

Examples of how to thin the thick fluids are given below.

POINTS TO THIN LIVER BLOOD

- Liv 14 (Front-mu, Liver).

- Liv 5 (Luo point, Liver).

ADVICE FOR PATIENTS

- Consume more water or thin fluids.

- Regular sports and exercise help the Liver Qi to circulate Blood.

POINTS TO THIN LUNG DAMPNESS:

- Lu 1 (Front-mu, Lung).

- Lu 7 (Luo point, Lung).

ADVICE FOR PATIENTS

- Inhale water vapour and drink more water.

- Breathing exercises, hot and cold baths and saunas help the Lung Qi to circulate and eliminate dampness.

Blood deficiency in traditional Chinese medicine does not mean that the patient has a low haemoglobin count. But iron, both in food and as a supplement, does help to improve Blood.

Blood deficiency can cause wind symptoms

Most skin diseases cause itching or irritation of the skin. This irritating factor is called wind. Normally, wind makes functional energy, helping the Qi and Blood to move and flow. This is a very important aspect of our Qi. But when wind is in excess, it could be pathogenic in nature and cause irritation.

Often this wind irritation can be of a wandering nature, not fixed to a specific area. In neurodermatitis the skin is typically very dry and rather pale, except on affected areas, which are flat, dry and reddish and move around very quickly.

This wind rises up and wanders around uncontrollably because of the deficiency of Blood. If the Blood can be tonified, the skin will become moist and calm. It is the wind that makes these patients restless and nervous.

- Ren 14 and UB 15 (to tonify yin and yang aspects of Heart).

- Sp 10, GB 39 and UB 17.

- Earth point of any organ that is Blood deficient, e.g. Lu 9, Liv 3, K 3.

ADVICE FOR PATIENTS

- Eat red meat and take an iron supplement.

1.2.2 Yin

Yin is the *amount of water and thin fluid* that irrigates an organ. A deficiency of yin will cause dryness of skin, with hardening, cracking, peeling and possible wrinkling. When the yin is inadequate to control the yang, yang hyperactivity may ensue, resulting, from time to time, in heat symptoms, such as redness and inflammation, hot flushes and burning skin with inability to sweat due to insufficient fluid. These symptoms tend to manifest more in the upper part of the body, as heat rises upwards. However, there may be some night-time sweating, as the yin is greater at night and during sleep.

Yin is also the *substance and the structure* of an organ. Without the continuous supply of Blood and fluid, the tissue will shrink or collapse. Recurrent heat or inflammation in a tissue can also cause this situation by consuming the yin fluid. An example would be the contraction and shortening of a tendon following recurrent tendonitis.

Dryness makes the skin hard and tense or leathery. Patients look strained and their face mask-like, as if they cannot relax. They need to use moisturizing creams soon after washing the skin, in order to retain the moisture.

Yin has the ability to cool the body, and a patient with yin deficiency will have skin that feels hot to the touch. In menopause, a woman will age quite suddenly, because this is a yin-deficient state. As the female hormones decrease, the yin of the Kidneys (the reproductive system) diminishes. As the Kidney yin stores water for the body, the body becomes dry as the yin decreases.

Yin deficiency causes heat

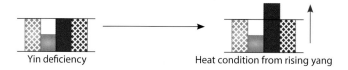

Yin deficiency   Heat condition from rising yang

The reproductive system is in the lower warmer of the Triple Warmer; the lung in the upper warmer. If the heat rises from the lower warmer, it will manifest in the upper warmer. Because the yin cannot control the yang, the heat or yang rises from time to time. As heat has an ascending nature, the heat that occurs in the reproductive system rises from the lower warmer to the upper part of the body, to the upper warmer of the three warmers. There are no real heat symptoms found in the lower part of the body (except perhaps hypermenorrhoea in post-menopausal and peri-menopausal women).

> A yin-deficient state causes a chronic latent heat condition in the organ. This could lead to recurrent phases of yang excess, each lasting for a short time. Some heat symptoms, however, will persist throughout the chronic period, e.g. a rapid pulse, red colour or red papillae on the tongue, low fever and red complexion.
>
> If the patient feels recurrent heat symptoms, but feels cold during the chronic phase and shows no other diagnostic signs of heat, then the patient also has a Blood deficiency together with yin deficiency.

Yin deficiency may cause stagnation of thick fluids

Yin deficiency and dryness can also affect the Blood and the thick fluid, by making it very thick and therefore difficult to flow. Thick mucus which cannot be expectorated easily will improve with damp (vapour) inhalation and drinking thin fluids. Similarly, if sebaceous secretion is very thick and cannot be easily eliminated, it would help to tonify both Kidney yin (for the water) and Lung yin (for the skin).

> Thick fluids tend to stagnate when they become too thick because of a yin deficiency. This would, in turn, lead to a Qi deficiency. When the yin is tonified, thick fluids flow easily and circulation and elimination improve.

- Drink thin fluids – water, herbal tea, clear soups and watery fruits.

- Some added salt in food (health permitting) to retain water.

- Some raw foods, especially vegetables (not in the evenings) to cool the body.

- Tonify Kidney yin – point K 7 or K 10.

- Tonify yin of affected organ – Front-mu point, own-element point of yin organ.

- Grandmother point of yang organ (e.g. St 43, wood point).

- If possible, take a nap around midday; this prevents the yang from attacking the body during its highest time in the day.

When the yin is good, the skin is smooth and elastic, soft and youthful. There are no small wrinkles.

If there is *water retention*, the skin could have a puffy appearance with some pitting oedema. This could be more evident in areas such as the eyelids, hands and neck, where the skin is thinner.

TREATMENT FOR YIN EXCESS

- Mainly with points and diet for increasing urination.

- UB 23 (needle and cupping), UB 58 and K 3.

- Cut down salty foods for at least the first half of the day.

> Yin deficiency causes *general dryness*, which should not be confused with *peripheral dryness*. If there is splitting of the fingertips or cracking of the heels, but the skin of the rest of the body is moist, this may be due to poor peripheral circulation of Blood. Peripheral Blood circulation is a Spleen function. It should be determined if this symptom occurs only in these areas.

1.2.3 Yang

Yang is the warmth that is brought on by good Blood and fluid circulation. This warmth helps to accelerate the function of the organs, without which they would slow down.

Yang deficiency

Yang deficiency causes coldness and clamminess of the skin. This is because coldness affects the function of the skin (Lung Qi) to open and close its pores when required, i.e. the skin pores should open, causing sweating and elimination of heat, when the body is hot; and should close and retain the body heat when it is cold. In this case, even though the skin is cold, the pores still remain open and there is some cold sweating.

Coldness on the skin causes it to be pale, but during activity or situations when the patient warms up, there will be a mixture of pink, blue and pale shades, causing a marbling effect on the skin.

Coldness could also be a symptom of Blood deficiency. If this is the case, the treatment would be to tonify the Blood (see page 26).

Yang excess

Inflammation and excessive heat or redness of the skin are all manifestations of a yang excess. Yang excess symptoms may be caused by inflammation, allergies or skin infections. Recurrent redness and inflammation may be a sign of either (1) yin deficiency and therefore quick rising of the yang (*fire heat* or *dry heat*) or (2) stagnation of dampness and festering heat from the dampness (*damp heat*).

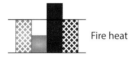 Fire heat   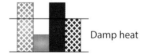 Damp heat

TREATMENT TO TONIFY YANG

- Moxibustion on Front-mu or Back-Shu point of organ.

- Tonification point or own-element point of yang organ of the coupled organs.

- Grandmother point of yin organ (e.g. Sp 1 wood point).

- Bitter foods, bitter teas.

- Red meat and fish.

- Eat cooked and warm foods; drink warm fluids.

EXAMPLE: TONIFY LUNG YANG

- UB 13 – Back-Shu point.

- LI 11 – tonification point of coupled yang organ.

- Lu 10 – fire point (grandmother point of Lung).

TREATMENT TO SEDATE YANG

- Blood-letting is a very effective way to reduce heat.

  - The points to bleed could be the Jing-Well point of the affected meridian, or the finger- or toe-tip of the affected meridian.

  - Plum-blossom hammer tapping to bleed affected area.

- Sedation point of yang meridian.

- SI 8 sedation; TW 10 sedation to reduce fire heat.

> The body uses bleeding as a way of eliminating excess heat. This occurs especially in situations in which the yin is deficient and therefore cannot control the yang. The only option is for the body to eliminate the yang, which it does by bleeding. Examples are epistaxis, excessive menstrual bleeding, vomiting of blood in patients with liver cirrhosis or gastric ulcer, bloody stool in patients with ulcerative colitis and coughing blood in patients with tuberculosis. When the body eliminates Blood, it has no control over the quantity of bleeding, so eventually there will be Blood deficiency. But we can use this principle, in theory, to eliminate heat without causing a Blood deficiency.

1.2.4 Qi

I use the word Qi (pronounced 'chee') here to mean function. The word Qi is used in many ways – to mean needle sensation (as in 'De Qi', which means that the energy has arrived), for breathing, for energy, for power, for anger, for working with energy, and so on.

I believe that the word Qi, when used alongside Blood, yin and yang, stands for function and movement. We can also talk about healthy Qi or function. Someone who needs to urinate every 15 minutes is suffering from hyperactivity of the bladder, which means that function is not appropriate. Healthy function is to be able to control urination depending on the quantity of urine in the bladder. If someone feels the urge to pass urine even though the bladder is nearly empty (as in nervous bladder) or if a person cannot pass urine when the bladder is full (as occurs in prostate enlargement), the bladder Qi is deficient (in both cases, it is not a healthy Qi).

Qi, as in function, has a yang nature – but it should not be confused with yang. It is true that climatic warmth activates organ function and cold slows it down. However, a pathogenic yang would actually inhibit organ function. For instance, the healthy digestive function of the stomach is affected during gastritis, and an inflamed joint suffers restricted mobility. Thus, it is evident that Qi and yang are not one and the same, although there are similarities.

In this book, the word Qi is always used to show function, movement and wind. Hyperactivity of an organ would indicate rising Qi (or excess Qi) and hypofunction would show it to be Qi deficient.

Each organ has its own function.

- Heart Qi synthesizes and circulates Blood and warmth, and governs mental activity and speech.
- Spleen Qi circulates Blood and fluid in the periphery, distributes nutrition, firms the connective tissue and senses taste.
- Lung Qi governs respiration, the opening and closing functions of the skin, the immune system and senses smell and touch.
- Kidney Qi governs water metabolism, the reproductive and the urinary system and senses sound.
- Liver Qi governs the storing and releasing of Blood in the vessels, generates wind for free flow of Blood, energy and fluid, controls muscles and tendons and senses sight.

Qi means function. In the case of the skin, it means the opening and closing function, which is important for adapting to temperature change. A patient whose Qi is deficient will feel very cold when there is a 2°C drop in temperature, and will feel very warm if the temperature becomes slightly warmer. Such individuals adapt reasonably well to weather that is constantly cold or warm, but changing temperature requires quick functioning of the skin. These patients tend to suffer from respiratory and skin problems, particularly during the changing seasons of the year (spring and autumn).

The functions of the skin are:
- To open the pores and eliminate heat, sweat and sebaceous secretion.
- To close the pores and hold in heat and fluid (especially sweat).
- Absorption (e.g. of nutritive creams applied externally).
- To participate in the immune system.
- Sensitivity to touch, pain and temperature.
- The firming of the skin, which depends not only on the skin, but also on the connective tissue that holds the skin firmly to the muscle – this is a function of the Spleen.

Factors that can affect skin function are:

- Cold, which closes the skin during winter and reduces the Qi.

- Pathogenic heat (inflammation), damp (from excessive damp-producing foods) and wind (chemicals that irritate the skin).

- Hot showers or baths in winter and exposure to cold weather.

- Poor skin hygiene (not cleaning or excessive make-up creams).

- Blood deficiency, which reduces the function because there is insufficient Blood to fuel functional energy.

Skin sensitivity is a sign of good function of the skin. When the skin is thick with thin or thick fluid, and therefore the yin aspect is comparatively greater than the yang, skin sensitivity is reduced. When we insert needles into our patients' skin, it is very noticeable that some patients are very sensitive to pain and some are not.

Those who have a thin skin (Blood deficient) or those who have a hot skin (yang excess) are generally more sensitive to pain or touch.

The principle of acupuncture analgesia is based on raising the pain threshold by either sedating the yang or tonifying the yin of the skin in the area of the surgery, so that patients feel less pain.

CHAPTER 2

SKIN TYPES

CHAPTER CONTENTS

Now that we have had a look at the concept of the Blood, yin, yang and Qi, let us examine the various skin types. We will continue with the visual representation of the four terms, as I believe that it is important for therapists to actually see the imbalance they are treating. This makes therapy very straightforward – the aim is simply to rectify any imbalance.

2.1 THIN AND DRY SKIN

 Blood and yin deficiency

The skin is thin, dry and pale, easily injured and slow to heal, with little or no body hair. When pinched at the forearm, it either feels thin like tissue paper (more Blood deficient) or hard like leather (more yin deficient). It will be hypersensitive to the sun or to pain, and would tend to have many small wrinkles on the thinner areas.

Possible causes of this state include:

- Not drinking water.

- A very low-fat diet.

- The absence of milk products in diet.

- A diet devoid of nutritious foods.

- Smoking.

- Malabsorption of nutrition due to diabetes mellitus or chronic diarrhoea (this is caused by either Small Intestine or Spleen Qi deficiency).

POINTS USED TO TREAT THIN AND DRY SKIN

- Lu 1, Sp 3 and K 10.

ADVICE FOR PATIENTS

In order to correct this, both Blood and thin yin fluids need to be tonified. Useful advice includes:

- Drink water frequently; some salt is required in the diet so that water is retained in the body.

- Consume milk products (especially buttermilk) and proteins, as well as grains and cooked root vegetables which are easy to digest and absorb.

- Watery fruits (melon, grapes, pears, etc.) are good for this condition.

- Some oil should also be used either in cooking, or raw in marinades and salads.

2.2 THICK, OILY AND RAISED SKIN

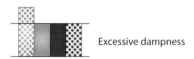

Excessive dampness

The skin will be thick in general, and can also be uneven and oily. Some areas could be raised compared with others, giving an island-like appearance. The skin is very greasy, and the sweat is thick, leaving marks on clothes. This is mostly in the face, neck and upper body. The lower part of the body is not usually affected in the same way, because the Lungs nourish the skin – and the Lungs are in the upper warmer area of the body.

Dampness originates in the Spleen, no matter where it manifests. Possible causes of Spleen dampness are:

- An excess of fatty foods.

- An excess of refined sugars or carbohydrates.

- An excess of fatty milk products.

- Large and heavy evening meals.

- An excess of cold and raw foods.

To rectify this, dampness should be circulated and eliminated.

POINTS USED TO TREAT THICK AND OILY SKIN

- Sp 9, St 40, UB 39, Lu 5 sedation.

- Sp 9 and St 40 are particularly useful.

- Avoid fatty foods and refined sugars.

- Eat only unrefined carbohydrates – sweet fruits, wholemeal bread and pasta, whole rice, millet, potato with skin.

- Take in few and low-fat milk products.

- Eat a good breakfast and lunch but have an early, light dinner.

- Drink warm drinks and eat only warm, cooked foods.

- Drink water regularly in order to liquefy the thick damp fluid.

2.3 THICK AND DRY SKIN

Stagnation of dampness and Qi deficiency

In this case, the skin is thick, uneven and even lumpy, but dry with seborrhoea on the surface. This means that there is fluid below the skin surface, but it does not ascend to the surface. The normal function of the skin is to bring fluid from under the skin to the surface. Therefore, thick and dry skin is a symptom of poor function of the Lung – that is, Qi deficiency.

The dampness stagnates under the skin, as it cannot be eliminated. This is a sign of poor ascending function of the skin, and not necessarily the descending function. However, it is possible that these patients are also constipated, as it is likely that there would be a problem in eliminating stools as well, because the Large Intestines are connected to the Lungs.

The avoidance of damp-producing foods is essential for treatment, but more important is to improve skin function (and bowel function) of elimination.

POINTS FOR TREATMENT

- Points to improve skin function – UB 13, LI 4 and LI 11.

- Points to improve bowel function – LI 4, TW 6, St 25.

- Points to reduce dampness – Sp 9, St 40.

- Keep your bowels open – take whole grains, apple or pears (including the skins) daily, and exercise to sweat.

- Whole rice should be eaten at least twice in a week – it strengthens the Lung yang and Qi.

- Take alternating hot and cold showers.

- Mild spices such as pepper and ginger should be added to the diet.

- Dress according to the climate – do not dress lightly in cold weather or overdress in hot weather.

2.4 THIN, DRY AND ITCHY SKIN

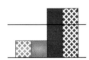

Blood and yin deficiency with wind-heat

Thin and dry skin is hypersensitive to heat or cold, sun, pain and allergens, and is therefore more likely to be itchy and irritated. This irritating aspect is called wind, and the redness caused by the manual scratching is the heat. As the Blood and yin are both deficient and therefore unable to control the wind and heat, the yang rises from time to time, bringing on recurrent wind-heat symptoms.

Treatment basically involves preventing this recurrent rise in the wind and heat by tonifying Blood and yin as in skin type 1 (see page 36). In addition, at acute times one could eliminate the heat and wind from affected areas.

There are excellent *wind-eliminating points*[1] all over the body, which should be used with wind-elimination sedation technique in this case:

- GB 20 – from head and face.

- UB 12 – from back, skin and lungs in general.

- SI 12 – from shoulders and arms.

---

1   Wind-eliminating points work best with the wind elimination needle technique (see page 103).

- GB 31 – from hips and legs.

- Ba Xie points – from hands.

- Ba Feng points – from feet.

For *heat elimination*,[2] it is possible to apply distal-point or fingertip bleeding, depending on the affected area. For example, in a case of eczema on the hands, fingertip bleeding on the affected meridian will bring about instant relief from both itching and inflammation.

Foods that aggravate wind symptoms include:

- Acidic foods such as vinegar-based pickles, tomatoes.

- Alcohol (particularly red wine).

- Citrus fruits such as lime, lemon, grapefruit.

- Foods that are common causes of allergic reactions, such as shellfish and other fish.

Foods that often cause heat reactions include:

- Red meat and red fish.

- Coffee and other caffeinated drinks.

2.5　THICK SKIN WITH INFLAMMATION OR PRURITUS

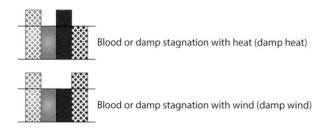

Blood or damp stagnation with heat (damp heat)

Blood or damp stagnation with wind (damp wind)

Damp heat condition of skin is common in acne vulgaris, furunculosis and varicose ulcers. The dampness manifests as thick, raised skin or as oedema, and stays fixed in one area. Heat originates from this fixed dampness in the form of inflammation or, if the skin is open, infection. The cause of the chronic inflammatory heat is the stagnation of damp, and therefore the therapy is to circulate, thin out and eliminate the thick fluid.

2　Heat-elimination needle technique (see page 102).

Blood stagnation – this would mean that there are either varicose veins or some obstruction in the venous blood flow causing blood stagnation and oedema. This results in Blood toxicity and heat (e.g. varicose ulcer or varicose eczema). In this case, treatment should be to improve venous circulation, which is more difficult to achieve than improving damp circulation.

Some ideas for treatment:

- Tonifying the Qi of the meridians along which the varicose veins are manifesting. If they are along the back of the leg, one could use UB 28, UB 58.

- Always tonify Liver Qi, as Liver is responsible for venous circulation: UB 18, GB 37.

- Point St 40 to improve the oedema.

In *Damp stagnation* the heat is localized to the damp areas and needs to be eliminated (if possible) from these areas. Treat dampness by:

- Thinning fluid (so it can flow) – drink water, K 10.

- Circulating fluid – St 40, UB 20 (needle and cupping), UB 39.

- Eliminating fluid – Sp 9, UB 23 (needle and cupping), K 3, UB 58 (through diuresis).

- Dispersing fluid – UB 13, LI 4, LI 11 (through sweating).

TO TREAT THE HEAT CAUSED BY EITHER BLOOD OR DAMP STAGNATION

- Plum-blossom needle tapping to bleed on the local areas.

- Finger- or toe-tip bleeding on affected meridians.

- Dispersing fire-needle technique on local acupuncture points.

Damp wind manifests as eczema (which is in fixed areas such as the neck, elbow, knee-fold and inguinal area), varicose eczema and functional itching in any area that is affected by oedema or is covered by clothes. It usually refers to itching confined to certain areas (a characteristic of damp), rather than itching all over or in different areas at different times (as in wind).

Wind is irritating in nature; thus, itching is a wind symptom. The symptom of damp wind shows that the wind is irritating the skin very close to its surface and needs to be eliminated by improving the skin function of opening the skin. The dampness is preventing the skin from functioning normally, and should therefore be circulated.

TREATMENT TO IMPROVE LUNG QI

- UB 13, LI 11, LI 4 (to open and eliminate).

TREATMENT TO ELIMINATE WIND

- Use wind-eliminating point of the area (see pages 39, 96, 99).

TREATMENT TO CIRCULATE DAMP

- St 40, UB 20, UB 39.

2.6 INFLAMED OR ITCHY SKIN

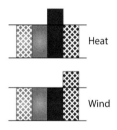

Heat

Wind

This situation is similar to the previous, except that there is no thick or raised skin and no oedema, and symptoms are not necessarily fixed in a specific area. The treatment, too, is for the heat only in the case of inflammation, and wind-eliminating points in the case of itching and wandering sites. The treatment of heat and wind are explained in the section on skin type 4 (page 39), and the same food restrictions apply as in skin type 4, against the heat and wind.

2.7 MIXED SKIN

Spleen Qi deficiency or Triple Warmer Qi deficiency

It is very common in people with skin problems for the skin to be oily in certain places and dry in others. Two patterns occur:

- *Oily skin on face and dry skin on legs.* This is a problem between the three warmers (San Jiao), where there is dampness stagnating in the upper warmer and yin deficiency in the lower. Treatment would be to descend the dampness from the upper and tonify the yin in the lower.

- *Patchy skin on the face, where one area is oily and another dry.* This is caused by poor distribution of dampness in the skin surface. Since peripheral circulation of dampness is a Spleen function, this would be a symptom of Spleen Qi deficiency.

TREATMENT OF TRIPLE WARMER QI DEFICIENCY

- UB 22, UB 39, Lu 5, Sp 6, K 7.

TREATMENT OF SPLEEN QI DEFICIENCY

- UB 20, St 40, Sp 1.

- Massage the skin surface with light moisturizer to improve circulation.

- When treating oily skin, some subcutaneous local needling helps.

- When treating dry areas, better results may be obtained by tonifying the yin of the organs in that area. For example, dry legs would benefit from Kidney yin tonification, point K 7; or dry arms with point Lu 9 or H 9.

CHAPTER 3

THE FIVE ELEMENTS AND THEIR ASSOCIATION WITH THE SKIN

CHAPTER CONTENTS

The *skin* has a complex relationship with the organs other than the Lung and cannot be singularly considered or treated. One by one, I would like to take you through the organs of the five elements (Figure 3.1) and their association with the skin.

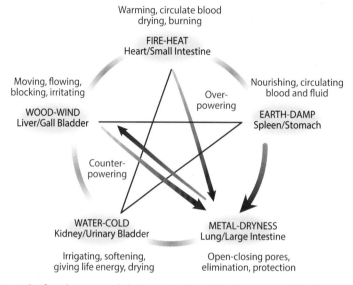

Figure 3.1 *The five elements and their association with the Lung and the skin*

3.1 FIRE – HEART AND SMALL INTESTINE

The Heart synthesizes and circulates Blood, which nourishes all the cells it reaches, and also warms the body. In other words, it improves the Blood and yang aspects.

The term Blood is used sometimes specifically to mean red blood, and is sometimes used loosely to mean nutrition. Blood provides tissues with not only oxygen and nutrition, but also fluid. If Blood does not reach an area, this area will be cold, malnourished and dry. This situation is common in skin diseases in the hands and feet, partly because these are often cold areas, and partly because circulation of Blood to these areas is generally poor.

The Heart and Lung are situated in the thorax, in the upper warmer, and they often influence the energy status of each other. Often the pulses are similar in the cun position (distal pulse position) of both wrists and symptoms in both organs – Lung/Heart and Small Intestine/Large Intestine – are comparable.

I would like to go deeper into the Blood, yin, yang and Qi of the Heart and, as this is also our first element, it will provide a good foundation for the elements to come.

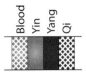

As you can see from the information in Table 3.1, the Heart and Lung are in the same area of the body; they influence each other by their proximity, they share the same secretion (Heart secretes sweat but the skin has to control the function of sweating) and their emotions are felt in the thorax.

According to the relationship between the five elements, the fire element has a controlling or overpowering relationship over the Lung, in the metal element. This means that excessive heat in the fire element would consume the yin in the metal element, making it dry and hot.

If the yang of the fire element were low, the lungs would become cold and wet without sufficient yang to control it.

TABLE 3.1 BLOOD, YIN, YANG AND QI

Blood	Yin	Yang	Qi
Red blood nourishes and oxygenates; when the Blood quantity is good, the complexion is evenly pink	There is a great amount of water or moisture in Blood; this cools and thins the Blood and cools upper body and hands	Warmth or heat in Blood, temperature of thorax, head and hands; when the yang is good, there is colour and shine on the face	Heart rate, circulation of Blood and fluid in the body also determine the heat in the upper warmer
Red blood provides continuous nutrition to the tissues of the body, and determines whether the 'evening face' is as fresh as the 'morning face'	Heart secretes sweat, and the fluidity of sweat depends on the Heart yin	Yang excess would manifest in a red face, perhaps with excessive sweating if the yin is also good	Heart Qi gives alertness to the mind and manifests in whether or not a person looks awake and alert
	Heart and Lung yin should irrigate the skin continuously, and the skin should remain moisturized throughout the day	The colour and shine of the facial skin would increase with activity or heat	The 'awake look' of an active Heart Qi is continuously nourished by Heart Blood
Blood deficiency causes paleness and coldness of the upper body. It also causes poor memory, insomnia and dryness, mostly of the upper body, and hands with cold sweating (normally, there should not be sweating in cold areas, but this is caused by a Blood deficiency bringing about a Qi deficiency)	Yin deficiency causes heat in the upper body with malar flush, fast heart rate, less and concentrated smelly sweat, anxiety and panic attacks and dream-disturbed sleep. As the heat has an upward disposition, the lower part of the body has a normal temperature or could even be cold	Yang deficiency mainly causes coldness and paleness of the upper warmer and hands, clammy skin, poor concentration and sleepiness. As coldness retards the opening and closing functions of the skin, the colder parts of the body are wet with sweat, though not excessively	Qi deficiency manifests in symptoms of poor circulation, concentration, slow mental function, bradycardia and arrhythmia. When bad, there could be cyanosis and oedema

Skin is often marbled between pale and blue colours; dry arms and hands; facial skin is dull, pale and lifeless	Skin is often hot, red and dry, and tense in chest, arms and hands	Skin is cold and clammy to touch, and the face is pale and without much expression	Qi deficiency often causes circulation problems where Blood does not reach certain areas in the extremities, especially the hands
Patient is usually depressed and uninterested, could also have constant sadness if lungs are weak, and weep all the time. But they want to have help	Face is red or with malar flush. Patient is restless, speaks fast and may have night sweating and could suffer from high blood pressure	Depression in cold weather; skin or lung diseases are aggravated by cold weather and improve when weather is warm	Skin diseases are of a fixed nature, with a thick, purple colour. There may be dryness on the surface, but with fluid below the surface
As Heart Blood deficiency often leads to Liver Blood deficiency, there may be overuse pains in tendons of the arms and small joints in hands	Skin diseases are usually of a hot nature, and occur on the thorax, arms or face and seldom in the lower part of body	Skin diseases occur more in the upper body and seldom in the lower	The upper part of the body is commonly affected but not below the level of the diaphragm

Excessive heat in Heart and Small Intestine

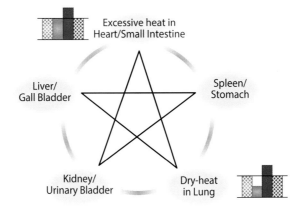

Figure 3.2 Heat in Heart and Small Intestine

An excess of Blood (Figure 3.2) and circulation create heat and redness of the skin, causing dryness and a burning feeling. The skin can become hard and leathery, and tense with less suppleness. These symptoms occur more in the upper part of the body, where both the Heart and Lung reside. The skin symptoms worsen in hot weather, or when feeling hot under bedcovers. Patients can suffer from hot flushes, burning skin with less sweating, mental restlessness and insomnia.

POINTS TO SEDATE HEART YANG TO COOL THE HEAT

- Sedate SI 8, TW 10.

- Sp 6 descending technique[1].

- Ren 14, H 5, P 6, Du 20 and K 7.

Coldness in Heart and Small Intestine

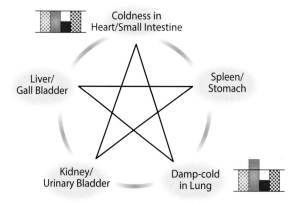

Figure 3.3 Coldness in Heart and Small Intestine

Deficiency in the Heart and Small Intestine yang will cause Lung yin and damp to be undercontrolled (Figure 3.3). This will make the entire skin cold and clammy, thick and oily. There will be much, thick, body hair, especially in men, because hair grows more on colder areas of the body which need more insulation – the chest and arms in this case. Patients may suffer with chronic cough or asthma with excessive mucus, and may be rather melancholic.

---

1   Descending technique on point Sp 6 is used to bring the heat down to the lower part of the body, away from the upper part. See pages 105–7 for the technique.

- UB 15, UB 13 (needle and cupping).

- SI 3, Lu 10, LI 6, St 40.

Heart Blood and Qi deficiency

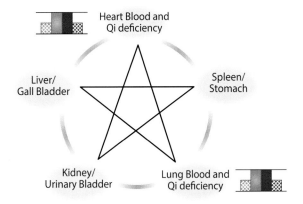

Figure 3.4 Heart Blood and Qi deficiency

A deficiency of Blood and Qi in the Heart causes paleness and cold, dry, dead-looking skin (Figure 3.4). The hands may also be blue or white, cold and sweaty – because the deficient Lung Qi cannot hold the sweat in. Patients are likely to suffer symptoms such as endogenous depression, anxiety, mental fatigue and sleep problems. If the Blood and Qi are tonified, the patient's mood, complexion, sleep and confidence all improve, and their skin glows pink with warmth.

POINTS TO TONIFY BLOOD AND QI OF HEART

- Ren 14, UB 15, Lu 1, UB 13.

- UB 17, Sp 10, GB 39.

ADVICE FOR PATIENTS

- Take Floradix – herbal iron formula for building Blood.

- Eat a nutritious diet.

3.2 EARTH – SPLEEN AND STOMACH

In the five-element relationship, the earth element (represented by the Spleen and Stomach) is the 'mother element' of metal (Lung and Large Intestine). This is the direct source of energy for the metal organs.

If the Spleen is Blood deficient (which in this case indicates a nutritional deficiency causing the patient to be thin or malnourished), then the Lung will become weak as there is no continued supply of nutrition. This causes the skin to be thin and vulnerable to damage, tending to injure easily and to heal poorly after injury.

Excess dampness in the Spleen (caused by excessive refined sugars and fatty foods in the diet) will make the skin thick and oily, with excessive and thick sebaceous secretions.

Excess thick fluid (with inadequate thin fluid to thin it down) will slow down the Qi of circulation of fluid and Blood in the periphery, thus also affecting the skin function (Lung Qi) of opening the pores and eliminating sebaceous secretions through the skin.

The Stomach receives and digests the food and drink we consume, and the Spleen absorbs and stores the nutrition, which is then used to nourish the Blood. This Blood is circulated throughout the body by the Heart, and to the periphery by the Spleen. It is the function of the Spleen to circulate Blood and distribute nutrition to the skin and the arms, legs and face.

Spleen Blood deficiency

Poor eating habits and malnutrition cause Blood deficiency in the Spleen and, as the Spleen nourishes the Lungs, in the Lungs and skin as well (Figure 3.5). The skin becomes thin, wrinkled and easily injured, and wound healing is delayed.

It is necessary to eat some damp-producing foods to fill the wrinkles in the skin. One 4 fl. oz cup of buttermilk a day will keep those million tiny wrinkles away!

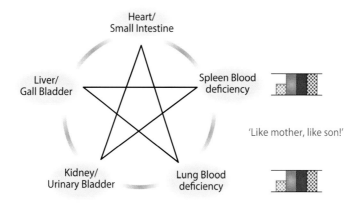

Figure 3.5 Spleen Blood deficiency

Patients with skin that injures easily and heals poorly need to eat more protein. Slow-cooked chicken soup, cooked with bones and vegetables for over 2 hours and consumed once daily, mung bean sprouts, lentils, and cooked and puréed pumpkin, butternut squash or potato soup (thick soups without fat but full of nutrition) are good foods to improve Spleen Blood.

The fact that food is cooked for a long time and is consumed warm will not only ensure that it is more easily digested and absorbed, but will improve the Spleen Qi and yang as well. The improved Spleen yang and Qi will circulate the Blood better in the periphery, thus transporting the nutrition to the skin and the extremities. Slow-cooked soups, stews and casseroles are good meals in winter, and when patients suffer from Spleen Blood and Qi or yang deficiency.

POINTS TO TONIFY SPLEEN AND LUNG BLOOD AND YIN

- Sp 3 (own element point).
- Lu 9 (tonification point).

ADVICE FOR PATIENTS

- Consume proteins and buttermilk.
- Eat slow-cooked and easy to digest foods.

Dampness in Spleen

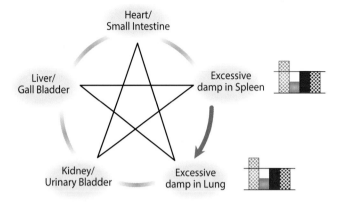

Figure 3.6 Dampness in Spleen

Excessive fatty foods, milk products, stodgy puddings, creamy sauces, refined carbohydrates and sugars, foods fried in oil and large evening meals cause dampness in the body and the skin (Figure 3.6). These foods should be avoided when the skin is thick and oily. Acne vulgaris (see page 132) is an example of such a skin condition, even though it has the additional complication of inflamed skin. Dampness is associated with thick body fluids, and foods of such consistency should be replaced by thin fluids, such as clear soups, watery fruits and unrefined carbohydrates and grains.

POINTS TO DISPERSE DAMPNESS IN SPLEEN AND LUNG

- Sp 9, St 40, UB 39.
- UB 13, UB 20, Lu 5.

ADVICE FOR PATIENTS

- Avoid fatty milk products.
- Avoid large late-evening meals as this is the lowest energy time for the Spleen and Stomach on the organ clock.
- Consume more fish, vegetables and unrefined carbohydrates.
- Consume cooked and warm drinks – preferably herbal teas and water.

Spleen Qi deficiency

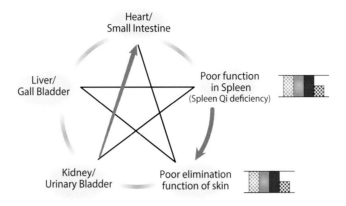

Figure 3.7 Spleen Qi deficiency

Spleen Qi ensures the even distribution of nutrition, especially in the periphery, and keeps the thick body fluids in constant circulation. A deficiency of Spleen Qi may cause stagnation of thick body fluids in different parts of the body (Figure 3.7). As fat tissue is also considered thick fluid, this could cause symptoms such as oedema of the eyelids, face or extremities, and cellulite.

Another very important function of Spleen Qi is that it firms the connective tissue of the body. Connective tissue is what attaches the skin to the muscles, thus giving the skin a firm appearance. When this becomes slack, the skin hangs away from the muscle, leading to the appearance of sagging.

> The Spleen Qi has a very important function in firming the connective tissue. The connective tissue holds the skin firmly to the muscle, giving it a wonderfully 'lifted' appearance. At the first sign of early ageing (around 35 years for women and 40 years for men), the earliest imbalance is that of decreasing Spleen Qi, and with that all the skin starts giving in to the forces of gravity!

POINTS TO TONIFY SPLEEN AND LUNG QI

- UB 13, UB 20 (Back-Shu points – improve the functional Qi).

- St 36 (own-element point).

- St 40 (Luo-connecting point).

- LI 4 (governs general elimination).

- LI 11 (improves Large Intestine function).

ADVICE FOR PATIENTS

- Eat warm and cooked food and drinks.

- Drink plenty of water and eat watery foods.

- Eat unrefined carbohydrates (especially millet and whole rice) and clear soups.

- Take regular saunas and exercise.

3.3   METAL – LUNG AND LARGE INTESTINE

The metal element consists of the Lung and Large Intestine organs. The Lungs govern both respiration and the skin; the Large Intestine is the great eliminator of the bowels and controls all elimination processes of the body.

Imbalances of the Lung can cause respiratory problems. This includes problems with the nose and sinuses.

For example, a blocked nose or excessive nasal discharge is because Lung dampness or yin is in excess, as would be the case with Lung oedema or a cough with excessive mucus. In these cases, the skin is in a similar state of imbalance – and is thick and oily or moist and sweaty. The same pattern of imbalance manifests in the Large Intestine also, resulting in semi-solid or watery stools.

If the Lung yin is deficient, this is manifested as dryness of the respiratory system (with dry cough, dry nose, etc.) and dry skin. In addition, the stools will be dry and there will be a tendency towards constipation.

Coupled organs have an interior–exterior energy flow. Therefore, they have the same picture of imbalance and similar symptoms. If there is a block between their interior or exterior energy flow, then they may have differing energy states. As their energy states are usually the same, the treatment is performed mostly on the yin organs to influence their yin, and on the yang organs to influence their yang.

As the metal element is the most important element for the skin and its wellbeing, let us take a closer look at the imbalances of the Lung and its coupled yang organ, the Large Intestine.

Lung yin deficiency

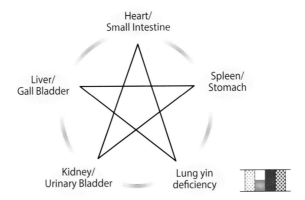

Figure 3.8 Lung yin deficiency

This means that the respiratory system and the skin are low in moisture (Figure 3.8). The skin will be dry and pale (white is the colour associated with metal, and any deficiency in the Lung tends to result in a pale facial complexion – a bright pale complexion in this case), with a tendency to crack and peel. The dryness causes a tight 'mask-like' effect, especially on the face. The body hair is nourished by the Lung, and there will now be less hair and it will be dry and rough without shine, turning a shade lighter.

As the Lung governs the respiratory system, dryness in the Lung will also result in a dry nose and throat and perhaps a dry cough. When the Lungs are dry, the Large Intestine, their coupled organ, does not receive sufficient yin from its yin partner – and also suffers from lack of moisture. This could manifest in constipation with dry stools, and anal fissure or haemorrhoids.

Of the organs of the five elements, the Lung and Large Intestine of the metal element are the most vulnerable to climatic dryness. A dry climate has less moisture. When we expose our body to climatic dryness (such as by using central heating in the winter months), it takes moisture away from the body. The parts of the body first affected by the dryness are the skin and the respiratory system. The stools may also become dry as the coupled organ is affected in the same way as the Lung.

Dryness causes a hard and rough skin that is often exacerbated or caused by Kidney yin deficiency, as the Kidneys irrigate the entire body. Over a longer period, dryness causes hardness or leatheriness of the skin. It refuses to absorb water. In the same way that water runs off a lotus leaf, dry skin also tends to lose water.

It has to be mentioned that dryness – as described here – refers to the skin surface. The skin can differ in thickness depending on its state of nutrition (from Lung Blood which nourishes the skin and Spleen Blood which nourishes the Lung) and both thick and thin skin can be dry on the surface. If thin skin is dry, this indicates a lack of fluid or water; thick skin has some fluid below the skin surface, so the dryness here is due to its inability to open the pores and let the fluid ascend to the skin surface.

Thin skin is often caused by a lack of nutrition and, just as a malnourished mother cannot breastfeed a baby well, poor skin nutrition is often due to poor nourishment (Figure 3.9). A good general state of nutrition results in a well-nourished skin. Foods that are particularly nourishing to the skin are those that nourish the Spleen as well: proteins, milk products, grains, root vegetables and slow-cooked stews to name but a few.

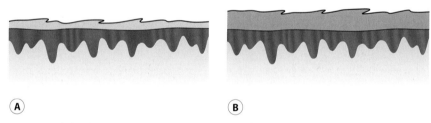

A   B

Figure 3.9 (A) Thin skin with a dry surface;
(B) thick skin with poor open–ascend function – dry surface

Points to tonify Lung yin

- Lu 1 – Front-mu point of Lung.

- Lu 8 – own-element point of Lung.

- Ren 17 – influential point of respiratory organs and skin, given in the direction of Ren meridian flow.

- K 10 – own-element point of Kidney, improves yin in entire body; it tonifies Kidney yin while also sedating Large Intestine yang.

- Drink water throughout the day and take some salt in the diet to help retain water.

- Humidify rooms and inhale water vapour.

- Use an aqueous cream after washing to hydrate the skin.

- Eat white rice at least twice a week.

Lung yin deficiency through Liver Blood deficiency

Liver Blood deficiency also can be a very important cause of dry skin. As Blood also nourishes and irrigates the skin, Liver Blood deficiency may manifest as dry skin and other symptoms such as paleness or marbling of skin, poor healing, hands and legs going to sleep easily, dizziness, scanty menstrual bleeding and blurred vision. Dry skin due to Liver Blood deficiency could be thin or thick. As Blood is more of a nutritional factor than an irrigating factor, Liver Blood deficiency tends to produce rather a thin skin in more cases.

> Dry skin could also be due to Liver Blood deficiency, and it is necessary to rule this out or treat this as well. Symptoms of Liver Blood deficiency include dry skin as well as brittle nails, extremities that go to sleep easily but improve with movement, dry eyes, tension and contraction in the tendons with a tendency for them to be inflamed with overuse, paleness, weak muscles and long menstrual cycles with scanty bleeding.

POINTS TO TONIFY LIVER BLOOD

- Ren 14, UB 15 (Front-mu, Back-Shu points of Heart).

- UB 17, Sp 10 (influential point of Blood/Sea of Blood).

- P 6, GB 39 (influential point for bone marrow).

- Liv 8 (tonification point).

It should be noted that the Heart Back-Shu and Front-mu points are used here to tonify Heart yin and yang, as Heart synthesizes Blood and Liver only stores and releases Blood.

Advice for patients

- A herbal iron substitute will be very useful in this case.

Thick skin is due to excessive dampness or stagnation of dampness. This normally goes together with Spleen dampness. Excessive dampness results from the consumption of damp-producing foods such as fats and fatty milk products, refined sugars and carbohydrates and late-evening meals; stagnation of dampness occurs for the same reasons but also because of insufficient physical exercise to produce Qi (to move the dampness). As dampness is thick fluid, the more thick fluid we have in our body and skin, the thicker it will become. And if the thin fluid dries out, the thick fluids will become even thicker in consistency, thus making it difficult for them to flow and circulate leading to stagnation. The thick fluid reduces the function of ascending and eliminating thin fluids to the skin surface, thus making the skin dry.

Lung yin deficiency causing Large Intestine yin deficiency

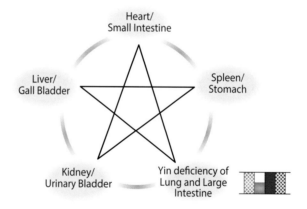

Figure 3.10 Lung yin deficiency and Large Intestine yin deficiency

Dry skin shows a yin deficiency of the Lung, and often there is a yin deficiency of the Large Intestine at the same time (Figure 3.10). Dry skin manifests in rough, peeling or cracking skin that is very painful (more so because there is a raised sensitivity as the yin is less and the yang is relatively higher), and the yin deficiency of the Large Intestine results in dry, hard stools, with straining potentially provoking haemorrhoids or anal fissures.

A yin deficiency is a chronic deficient state from which there could be recurrent episodes of rising yang excess. Both Lung and Large Intestine yang could rise from time to time, producing inflammation of the skin or Large Intestine. Symptoms such as acute recurrent chest infections or colitis could occur. The mucous membranes, skin and the intestinal flora are hypersensitive to pain, heat, strongly flavoured food and even emotional changes. These would be the causative factors for the aggravation of the recurrent episodes.

POINTS TO TONIFY LARGE INTESTINE YIN

- St 25, LI 5.

- K 10 – own-element point of Kidney, improves yin in entire body; it tonifies Kidney yin while sedating Large Intestine yang.

ADVICE FOR PATIENTS

- Drink water throughout the day.

- Take some salt in the diet to retain water.

- Eat white rice at least twice a week.

Lung yin deficiency causing intermittent heat excess or wind-heat excess

As yin naturally controls yang, a deficiency of the yin means that the yang can be undercontrolled, and can rise from time to time. This would bring about heat or wind-heat symptoms of the skin, such as inflammation, itching or burning. A heat rash could appear, manifested mainly by flat areas of red skin or pimples, only a few of which contain pus. There is little thick sweat or no sweat, but there may be more night sweating – as night-time and sleep can increase the yin of the Lung.

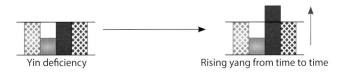

Yin deficiency   Rising yang from time to time

Yin tonification is the key to treating a chronic, recurrent heat condition on dry skin. The heat can be eliminated at the time it manifests, but if the yin is not tonified, the condition will reoccur.

- If there are specific areas that are dry, yin tonification points on these areas could be used, e.g. for dry palms use P 8 and for dryness in the popliteal fold use UB 40.

POINTS TO TONIFY LUNG QI

- LI 4, UB 13, LI 11 (help ascend and disperse fluid from below skin level to surface).

WAYS TO ELIMINATE HEAT OR WIND-HEAT

- Wind-heat – this will be manifested as redness and itching areas appearing quite suddenly, which are of a wandering nature.

  ○ Use wind-eliminating points for the affected area with the wind elimination sedation technique (see page 105).

  ○ Foods that cause wind-heat such as alcohol, pickled foods, citrus or sour-flavoured fruits and tomatoes should be avoided.

- Heat without itching.

  ○ Use any acupuncture point in the affected area, with the heat-dispersing technique (see page 102)

  ○ Use venous bleeding on a local or distal point (e.g. Lu 5).

  ○ Use finger- or toe-tip bleeding on the affected meridian.

  ○ Use plum-blossom tapping to bleed locally.

  ○ Avoid foods that cause heat such as red meats and shellfish. Coffee and bitter-flavoured teas and spicy food should be avoided.

POINTS TO SEDATE HEAT OF LARGE INTESTINE

- Sedate point LI 2 (sedation point).

- Sedate point St 37 (lower sea point of Large Intestine).

- Use heat-elimination needle technique on point UB 25 (Back-Shu point).

- Sp 10, LI 11 and UB 17 can be used in cases of wind and heat and also in the interval period to cool and purify the Blood.

Dampness in the Lung

Dampness in the Lung originates predominantly from the Spleen; the Spleen dampness is mostly (but not only) caused by damp-producing foods. Symptoms will be thick, oily skin that looks unclean with spots and pimples. These pimples may get infected easily and form pustules. When these pimples and pustules heal, they leave deep scars, making the skin look uneven.

This appearance of the skin seems to occur more in the regions of the face, neck and front and back of the thorax, and the lower part of the body is seldom affected. These are the areas associated with the upper warmer, which the Lung governs, and this may be why the skin on the lower part of the body is not affected so much.

There are, however, two points to note when treating dampness anywhere in the body.

An excess state with an excess of dampness in the interior

There is *excessive thick fluid*, which means there is an excess state. This is often caused by a diet high in fatty and milky foods, foods cooked in oil and refined sugars as well as large quantities of rich foods. There is also a stagnation of this dampness, which is not distributed through the entire body, but stays in the upper body and just under the skin. The Spleen Qi, which should be circulating this dampness evenly throughout the body, does not seem to be functioning well.

In this situation, the Large Intestine would generally be affected in a similar fashion, with semi-solid stools tending to be yellow-brown coloured. There can also be abdominal distension and pains.

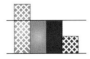

Stagnation of excessive dampness with Qi deficiency in the Spleen

POINTS TO TREAT EXCESSIVE DAMPNESS IN LUNG

- Sp 9, St 40, UB 20 – eliminate and circulate Spleen dampness.

- UB 13, LI 4 and LI 6 – eliminate dampness from skin.

- UB 39 – will help in distributing dampness in the Triple Warmer.

- Superficial local needling will help to circulate damp in the areas where there is stagnation.

- Avoid damp-producing foods.

- Turkish baths or saunas will help to open skin pores.

The thick fluid is too thick and gluey (because of insufficient yin)

The thick fluid is too thick because the yin (the thin fluid within this thick fluid) is deficient. This makes the consistency of the fluid too thick to circulate or to be eliminated from the skin. Moreover, the scars from all the old pimples remain hard and deep, and the skin does not return to its normal softness and remains hard and uneven in these areas. This hard, thick fluid also clogs the skin pores with a talcum-like formation and further worsens the elimination function of the skin.

Here, the stools tend to be hard and darker coloured, indicating the dryness. The patient will be more constipated for long periods, without an urge to defecate.

Thick fluid becomes thicker and more solid because the yin is deficient – this affects the circulation and elimination functions of the thick fluid.

POINTS TO TREAT DAMPNESS WITH YIN DEFICIENCY

- Lu 1, K 10, Ren 17 (to tonify Lung yin).

- UB 13, LI 4 and LI 11 (will improve the elimination function).

ADVICE FOR PATIENTS

- Drink more water.

- Moisturize the skin.

- Humidify rooms to tonify Lung yin.

- Steam baths will help to open skin pores.

Wind invasion of Lung (Liver wind attacking the Lung)

Generally this means that the wind – an exterior climatic factor – attacks the body from outside, and causes skin aversion and irritation to wind (manifesting in goose pimples). It can also enter the upper respiratory system through the nostrils and cause sneezing, a blocked nose, headache, sinusitis and pharyngitis.

But, in skin diseases, *wind is often generated in the interior of the body* – it is not an exogenous pathogenic factor. Wind is generated by the Liver, and when the Lung yin (which should overpower the Liver yang or Liver wind) is too weak, the Liver wind acts counter to the Lung, irritating the skin and the respiratory system and causing itching, sneezing and other symptoms associated with an allergic reaction. Also, the skin lesions move around without having a fixed locus, as is the character of wind.

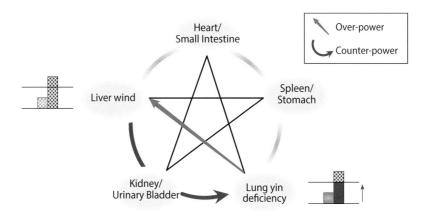

Figure 3.11 Wind invasion in the Lung

Figure 3.11 shows Lung yin too weak to control Liver yang and wind. Liver wind counter-powers the Lung (attacks the Lung against the direction of the normal controlling cycle), and causes wind symptoms of the Lung and skin – Liver wind invades the Lung.

POINTS TO TREAT WIND INVASION OF LUNG

- GB 38 sedation (sedates Liver wind and yang).

- Tonify Liv 5 (tonifies Liver yin).

- Ren 14, UB 15, Sp 10, UB 17 and GB 39 (tonify Liver Blood).

- Lu 1, Lu 8 (tonify Lung yin, in order to reinforce control on wood).

- Use wind elimination points in the affected areas with the sedation technique.

ADVICE FOR PATIENTS

- Avoid sour, citrus and acidic foods and alcohol, which increase Liver yang.

Why does increased Liver wind attack only the Lung? Why does it not affect the Heart, Stomach or Intestines?

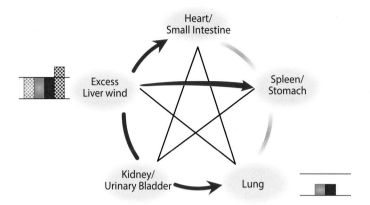

Figure 3.12 Excess Liver wind

As you can see from Figure 3.12, excess yang or Qi in an organ can flow in many directions. However, *energy always flows from areas of high energy to areas of low energy*. Therefore, excess Qi flows to where the yin or Blood is weakest. In this case, the Lung yin is weak and the yang is not high, so the excess Liver wind flows to the Lung, attacking the Lung yin further and causing wind symptoms in the Lung areas of the body. It is also possible, for example, for the Stomach yin to be weak, so that the Liver wind flows to and irritates the Stomach.

When the skin needs the wind

Wind is necessary for Blood, energy and body fluid to circulate. Just as an excess of wind will cause irritation to the skin and wandering skin lesions, a lack of wind will cause the skin lesions to stagnate, become thick and fixed and remain forever in areas which are not ventilated. Some patients improve in a seaside climate with sea breeze and salt water, not to mention the sun. With the warmth of the sun, the fluid or dampness lessens through osmosis from the salty water and the wind moving this blocked energy and dispersing it. What a tonification for the yang and the Qi! As the dampness reduces from the interior and under the skin, the damp sea breeze moisturizes the skin surface, softening it and thus helping its supple movement.

But it is not always possible for patients to go to a sunny seaside climate. At these times, they rely on the Liver to generate this warm wind. If the Liver yang and Qi are weak, there is less Qi to move around the blocked damp areas that are fixed at the folds and covered places of the body. It then becomes necessary to tonify Liver Qi and circulate and ventilate the damp areas.

- UB 18 and GB 37 (Luo) for Liver.
- UB 13 and LI 6 (Luo) for Lung.
- St 40 for circulating dampness in general.

ADVICE FOR PATIENTS

- Practise soft and harmonious exercises such as Qi Gong or Tai Qi.

Cold in the Lung

To feel warmth on the skin surface is an indication that there is good Blood flow to the skin. But when there is Liver Blood deficiency or when there is poor Blood circulation (Lung yang deficiency), the skin becomes cold (Figure 3.13). Skin conditions of a cold nature are vitiligo and psoriasis, which improve in the summer and with sunshine.

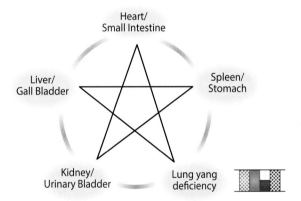

Figure 3.13 Cold in the Lung

Skin pigmentation generally increases with sunlight. People living in warm climates are usually dark skinned. Skin becomes depigmented when the yang descends to below skin level, leaving the surface with yang deficiency.

Similarly, psoriasis, which worsens in winter and in areas where there is less free flow of Blood (such as elbows and knees), improves in the summer and with sunshine.

Cold in the Lung can also cause respiratory problems such as asthma or chronic bronchitis, worsening in winter and improving in warm weather. There could be white and foam-like mucus and cold, clammy skin. The stools can be light-coloured and semi-solid.

Points to tonify Lung yang

- Moxa on UB 13, UB 15 and UB 17, with hot needles (the Lung is a large organ and it needs more Back-Shu points to influence it). This treatment is useful in problems of the organ, but not for the skin.

- Lu 10, LI 11 (tonify yang of Lung and Large Intestine).

- SI 3, TW 3 (tonify the yang of the fire element, so it can supply more yang to the Lung on the controlling cycle).

- In the case of vitiligo, psoriasis or other cold diseases of the skin, *ginger moxa* can be used on the local areas until the skin becomes red. Alternatively, use a *plum-blossom hammer* with light tapping, so as to cause a red skin reaction. These therapies ensure Blood flow to the affected areas, thereby improving the warmth.

Lung Qi deficiency

The function of the skin is to protect the interior of the body and the muscles and tendons from injury by exterior climatic factors. A healthy skin is soft and elastic, with quick opening and closing functions in order to keep in or let out body heat, as the situation demands. It should also be able to expel or retain sebaceous secretions, and keep the skin surface moist and shiny.

When the skin is too thin, it is hypersensitive to climatic factors, and will not be able to protect the interior sufficiently well. The body is very sensitive to heat, cold or wind, which can easily attack the interior.

A Large Intestine that has a yin deficiency will also be hypersensitive to foods and is easily irritated, giving rise to urgent watery and explosive stools.

When the opening and closing functions of the skin are affected in Lung Qi deficiency, it does not open its pores when necessary (i.e. when it is hot) nor does it close its pores when needed (i.e. when it is cold) (Figure 3.14). This could mean that when someone is hot, they cannot sweat to disperse the heat, but carry the heat to the interior instead. In these cases, patients complain of a burning feeling on the skin with no possibility of cooling it down.

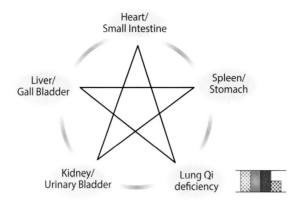

Figure 3.14 Lung Qi deficiency

Another symptom of Lung Qi deficiency is that someone who is cold will sweat excessively, especially in the colder parts of the body, thus becoming even colder. And because the opening and closing functions are slower than normal, there is poor adaptation to temperature changes in the climate. A person suffering from Lung Qi deficiency would feel very cold if the temperature dropped by 2°C, or feel very hot if the temperature increased by 2°C. They would, however, adapt better if the temperature remained steadily cold or hot. It is during the changing climates of spring and autumn that they seem to suffer most.

The Large Intestine that is confused as to when to open or close goes through phases of constipation and diarrhoea, and not always for logical reasons. Irritable bowel syndrome is a good example of this condition.

TREATMENT

- Points to treat thin skin are discussed on page 58.

POINTS TO TONIFY LUNG QI

- UB 13 (Back-Shu point).

- LI 11 (tonification point and a good immune-enhancing point).

- LI 4 (can be used where sweating is difficult, to open the skin).

- Lu 7 (can be used where there is excessive sweating, to close the skin).

- Take alternating hot and cold showers.

- Have a regular skin massage.

- Take a sauna in the winter months when the skin function becomes poor.

POINTS TO TREAT FOR THE LARGE INTESTINE

- St 25 and St 37 (to help Large Intestine function).

- LI 4 and TW 6 (to activate the Large Intestine function).

- LI 5 and K 10 (to soften the stools).

- St 25, Ren 4, Ren 12 and St 36 against bloating.

> When treating Lung or skin disease, it is advisable to look for blocks on the meridian. An external scar cutting across the meridian or an internal nodule, quite often felt at the radial styloid (near point Lu 8), can obstruct the flow of the meridian, thus causing an excess or deficient situation at one end of the block. The unblocking can be achieved simply by placing two needles – one proximal and one distal to the block – on the Lung meridian, and leaving it for 20 minutes along with other points used during treatment. This should be performed at least eight times to be effective in unblocking.
>
> Similarly, abdominal scars should be unblocked when treating bowel problems.

3.4 WATER – KIDNEY AND URINARY BLADDER

The Kidneys give water and life energy to all the tissues of our body. Kidney yin stores water for the body and Kidney yang irrigates the body with this water.

Water softens tissues and removes hardness. Skin that holds moisture in will be soft and supple, which will make the opening and closing functions more efficient. The body hair, which is moistened by the water, will be shiny and soft.

Kidney yin deficiency

A deficiency of Kidney yin means that there is less water for the whole body (Figure 3.15). There will be general dryness, and the urine will be concentrated and dark. There may be Kidney stones.

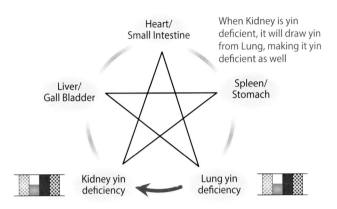

Figure 3.15 Kidney yin deficiency

If the Kidney is yin deficient, it will draw yin from the Lung, its mother organ. Over a period of time, this will cause a yin deficiency of the Lung, resulting in dryness of skin, nose, throat and stools. A good example of this combination of symptoms is post-menopausal syndrome.

Menopause is said to be a decline in female hormones and, as the reproductive system is governed by the Kidneys, this decline in hormones also means that there is a Kidney yin deficiency. One of the early symptoms of menopause is dryness of the skin, hair and many other areas. This causes wrinkling, hair loss, tiredness and intermittent heat symptoms (the heat symptoms are because the deficient yin can no longer control the yang). A woman who remains reasonably young-looking throughout her life will suddenly age from the time of her menopause. Women with Kidney yin deficiency may suffer from short menstrual cycles and excessive bleeding at the time of peri-menopause. This is because the Kidney yang rises from time to time, and the body eliminates the excessive yang through bleeding. As the yin is weak and therefore cannot rise to control the yang, this will be the only way for the body to balance the situation. Osteoporosis is also a sign of Kidney yin deficiency.

It is not just menopausal women who appear to age. People of any age or gender may become deficient in Kidney yin, and for various reasons. The principal reason is that people do not drink enough water. Often they don't drink at all, but sometimes they drink excessive tea, coffee and alcohol. Unfortunately, these are all diuretics, which increase urination and cause dryness and heat in the body (alcohol causes heat in the Liver, and tea and coffee cause heat in the Heart and both can increase Stomach heat).

Drinking water regularly throughout the day is important for improving Kidney yin. Herbal teas such as chamomile or green tea are also good for this purpose. It is necessary to sip water throughout the day, rather than drinking 2 litres of it whenever remembered. This will only lead one quickly to the toilet! Also, cooking in water (boiling, steaming, broiling, soaking) are better methods of enhancing water energy than baking, frying, roasting or microwaving.

The Kidneys store vital essence when we rest and make vital energy when we work. Just as a car consumes petrol, we use up our vital essence all through our active time. It is therefore necessary to occasionally rest and refuel. As work becomes more demanding and rest time becomes less, the Kidney yin is reduced. To punctuate the day with short periods of rest will help recovery. The best time for rest during the day is midday, the time of the highest yang. This is not always a practical solution for everyone, but doctors, the middle-aged and those who are self-employed or retired could practise this lifestyle.

Kidney yin and the water in the body are easily affected by exterior heat. Those who are deficient in Kidney yin should avoid direct exposure to the sun and avoid heat so that the yin will not be further consumed. People who live in tropical countries frequently carry an umbrella to protect them from the sun, and yet when people from Europe visit such countries they consider it safe to go out in the sun protected only by sun block. Sun and heat can injure the yin – not only of the skin but of the entire body, especially if there is pre-existing weakness of the yin.

Finally, some people drink lots of water but do not seem to retain any of it. They pass large volumes of urine, usually just after drinking water. This could be a Qi deficiency of the Kidney – where the Kidney is confused by when to hold water in the body and when to eliminate it. If this problem is not precipitated by caffeinated drinks, then it may be useful for sufferers to try increasing their salt intake.

> There is a popular belief among people that salty foods are unhealthy. According to the theory of the five elements, all foods in their natural form (this does not mean that food should be raw, but that it should not be modified or artificial), all flavours (again in their natural form – sweet fruit, for example, is better than sugar), all emotions (when not suppressed but felt and dealt with) and all colours (again natural and not intensified as they are in the television) are good – *in moderation*. When there is an absence or excess of one, then the problems begin.

Why, then, is salty food good in moderation? Because salt helps to hold water in the body, especially when the patient has large dry areas in the body – such as the skin and the mucous membranes – and the patient drinks enough fluids. Often these patients suffer with frequent urination following consumption of fluids, showing that they have problems with retaining water. If they are not on diuretics, or not suffering from hypertension, then it would be useful if they use a moderate amount of salt in their cooking. Sea salt is the better choice in this case.

An excessive amount of salt, however, will harden the blood vessels and cause water retention. It will also cause a dry mouth and excessive thirst.

Chronic Kidney yin deficiency leads to an intermittent increase in Kidney yang. If there is an increase in the yang, the body tries to balance this by increasing the yin. An example of this is feeling hot and sweating excessively. But when the yang rises on the basis of yin deficiency, then the only way the body can balance this situation is by eliminating the yang – which the body does by bleeding excessively from the heat source. If the patient was a woman of menstruating age, this would result in heavy menstrual bleeding.

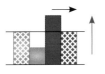

Kidney yin deficiency causes yang to rise, and the body eliminates the excess yang through bleeding

Due to the excessive bleeding, there could be a Liver Blood deficiency, which improves in the intervals between menstrual bleeding

As you can see from the above towers, the excessive bleeding will then lead to eventual Blood deficiency, which will in turn worsen the dryness.

POINTS FOR TREATING KIDNEY YIN TONIFICATION

- K 10 or K 7 (K 7 is not the best point in this case because it draws energy from Lung and makes the skin even drier; K 10 would be more suitable as this draws energy from Large Intestine yang).

- K 4 – this point is especially good in those with heat conditions, including excessive menstrual bleeding and hot flushes.

- GB 25 – Front-mu point of Kidney.

ADVICE FOR PATIENTS

- Drink water throughout the day.

- Use water in cooking; pre-soak grains and kidney beans overnight before cooking.

- Eat fish with white flesh.

- Have a midday rest.

- Have baths instead of showers.

- Take up swimming and spend as long as possible in the water.

- Cook meat with bones and make stock with bones – this is especially good for patients with osteoporosis.

When improving Kidney yin and Blood with these methods mentioned above, the Lungs and the skin improve automatically because the Kidneys are no longer deficient and do not rely on the lungs as their only source of water and nutrition.

Kidney yang deficiency

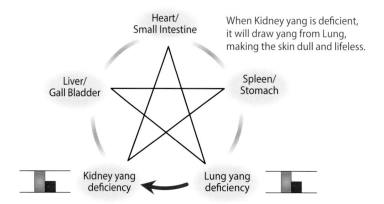

Figure 3.16 Kidney yang deficiency

Kidney yang provides us with vital energy and life energy. When comparing two persons – one in their twenties and the other in their sixties – it is clearly evident that they are very different in their appearances, body language and energy states. The older of the two will be slower, with limited movements, dull and wrinkled skin with some liver spots, and with less and grey head hair. The younger person has more life energy, a youthful shiny skin, a good head of hair, more bounce in their step and more flexibility in movement. It is this 'bounciness' of the youthful state that the Kidney yang provides to our lives. Kidney yang brings more energy into our lives, more interest, more libido and more activity (Figure 3.16).

Kidney yang also brings warmth, especially to our bones and joints and to our legs and back. It makes the urinary system and the reproductive system function well. It livens up the condition of the head hair and makes the hearing acute. The Kidney yang is at its peak when our vital energy is at its highest. Figure 3.17 shows the peak times of vital energy and reproductive energy in men and women.

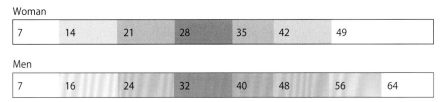

Figure 3.17 Peak times of vital energy and reproductive energy in men and women

> When Kidney yang is deficient, it will draw yang from the Lungs, making skin dull and lifeless.

If we treat patients in this age group to improve their youthful appearance, we will have nature on our side and the therapy will be very effective. But when we treat those whose vital energy is declining (most patients who come for cosmetic acupuncture!) then we will have to work harder and the patients will have to cooperate with us in maintaining their energy state and undergo further treatment periodically to maintain the energy balance.

So how does one activate one's Kidney yang? Unlike Kidney yin, which is mostly dependent on continuous water supply to the body, the Kidney yang depends partly on sportive physical activity and a healthy sexual activity. By this I mean that these should also be in moderation and not overly consuming. Extreme physical exercise and sex can deplete Kidney yin and Blood. Absence of exercise and sex will cause Kidney yang deficiency, which will further inhibit the interest in and ability to perform sex or physical exercise. Have you noticed someone in love? They are beaming from head to toe and have a body language boasting vitality and confidence. Those who indulge in regular physical exercise also show a wellbeing and youthfulness that cannot be bought with creams and massages.

In women of menstruating age, regular menstrual cycles and trouble-free periods are a good way of maintaining a healthy Kidney yang. If there are menstrual problems, then treating these will bring about an improvement in Kidney yang.

Kidney yang is attacked by overexposure to cold, especially on the lower parts of the body. Patients should be encouraged to keep their back and legs warm and avoid cold feet. Those with cold feet should have warm foot baths every evening so that they go to bed with warm feet.

Someone with good Kidney yang will look young and will have shiny skin and shiny, bouncy hair, twinkling eyes and rosy cheeks. When the Kidney yang is deficient, the skin and hair is dull, the face grey and lifeless and the eyes dull and reflecting lack of interest; the general appearance is of a lack of life force in that person. Even someone who is only 30 years old will look old and dull.

Moreover, Kidney yang deficiency causes many other symptoms, for example:

- The hair will become prematurely grey.

- The Urinary Bladder yang on the back may be weak, resulting in a hunched appearance as the yang on the back is not firm enough to maintain an upright posture.

- These patients may be lazy and have a low libido, which makes them less active and results in insufficient Qi to move Blood and fluids in the body.

- These patients may suffer with anxiety and phobias and their fears make them more passive and frustrated.

- They may suffer from water retention and oedema that increase during the day and improve overnight.

- Kidney yang deficiency can result in increased night-time urination, which disturbs sleep and makes patients feel tired during the day.

- It is quite a common problem in colder countries because of prolonged exposure to cold weather.

When the Kidney becomes yang deficient, it also draws energy from the mother organ, the Lung. As a result, the Lung can become yang deficient, causing dull skin and body hair, cold and clammy skin and a poor immune system. The Qi of the Lung and the skin function can slow down.

POINTS TO TONIFY KIDNEY YANG

- UB 23 (Back-Shu point).

- K 3 (the earth point or the grandmother point).

- UB 67 (tonification point of coupled yang organ, Urinary Bladder).

- Both LI 11 and St 36 can increase the yang in their organs and allow more yang to come into the Kidney through the mother–son cycle and the controlling cycle.

The first two points are the best to use in this case, because the UB 67 point will draw energy away from the Lung and Large Intestine, which will be deficient. But K 3, the earth point, will draw yang from the Stomach.

ADVICE FOR PATIENTS

- Partake in regular and moderate exercise, especially involving the back and legs. Cycling is a good sport for this.

- Eat red fish, shellfish, red kidney beans and cooked chicken feet or pig trotters (the feet of animals have Kidney yang energy because they are in the lower part of the body, and because they are an active part of the body).

- Have a foot massage or warm foot bath regularly.

3.5 WOOD – LIVER AND GALL BLADDER

The wood element is represented by the Liver and Gall Bladder organs. As with all the other elements, the organs of the wood element are also a very important influence on the Lungs and skin (Figure 3.18).

Like the Heart, the Liver has a close association with Blood – the Heart synthesizes Blood and the Liver stores and releases Blood. Blood here means red blood, which carries oxygen and nourishes and irrigates all tissues and the skin. Like Heart Blood deficiency, Liver Blood deficiency also causes paleness, dizziness and coldness. But there are some small differences between the two. See Table 3.2 for a comparison.

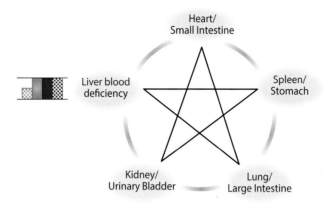

Figure 3.18 Liver Blood deficiency

TABLE 3.2 COMPARISON BETWEEN HEART BLOOD
DEFICIENCY AND LIVER BLOOD DEFICIENCY

Heart Blood deficiency	Liver Blood deficiency
Paleness, coldness and some dryness, especially in the upper part of body	Paleness and dryness all over the body
Mental fatigue, poor concentration and memory, poor sleep, depression, weak voice, breathlessness, palpitations, cold sweating, especially of hands (these symptoms of Qi and yang deficiency occur due to Blood deficiency)	Dizziness, dry eyes and blurred vision, easily numbed extremities but improving with movement, long menstrual cycles with scanty light-coloured bleeding, dry skin, dry head hair, loss of head hair, brittle nails, weak muscles and tendons, irritable when stressed
Pale tongue or pale at tip, empty pulse	Tongue pale on sides and there may be less coating on sides; empty, wiry pulse
Treatment	
Ren 14, UB 15, UB 17, GB 39, Sp 10, iron supplement	Same points plus Liv 8

The Heart synthesizes red blood and circulates it for the entire body, whereas the Liver stores and releases Blood from the Blood vessels, assuring the Blood flows without stagnation. If the Heart synthesizes less Blood, the Liver will have less Blood to store. Therefore, when treating Heart or Liver Blood deficiency, it is first necessary to tonify the Heart, in order to improve Blood synthesis, and thereby the Blood quantity.

Liver Blood deficiency

Liver Blood deficiency is common in cosmetic and skin problems. The skin will be dry all over and both body hair and head hair are sparse and in a poor state of malnutrition. The skin rarely has one colour, and generally looks marbled between pink, blue and pale shades. The eyes look sunken and dry and the muscles and tendons will be weak, causing hyperextension of the joints. The person lacks power and looks exhausted and irritable. These patients come for a pampering when they come for treatment, and no amount of face lifting will help them to look fresh and young, although energy treatment will.

I tell these patients that it is more important to treat their energy than their face. As cosmetic treatment is more expensive, four ordinary sessions are first carried out to build up the Blood and energy, following which cosmetic treatment will be very successful.

> When I perform a cosmetic acupuncture session, I devote the first 20 minutes to energy-balancing therapy. This makes the treatment more effective and longer lasting. But in the case of severe Liver Blood deficiency, I think it is better that no face lifting is done for the first four sessions. The patients arrive with high expectations, and we have to deliver! We cannot do this if their general energy state is too low. So we compromise, explain the reasons to the patient and build a good foundation to work on.

POINTS FOR TONIFYING LIVER BLOOD DEFICIENCY

- Ren 14, UB 15, Liv 8.

- UB 17, Sp 10, GB 39.

- Iron supplement (I normally recommend Floradix – herbal iron formula).

- Ren 6, St 36, Sp 6 and Lu 9 can be taken to improve general energy.

- GB 34 can be used if muscles and tendons are very weak.

Liver yin deficiency and Liver-fire

Liver yin stores Blood within the Liver and the Blood vessels and Liver yang releases Blood for the use of all organs. When the Liver yin is deficient, it does not hold the Blood in the vessels and there may be delayed coagulation in the case of an injury. We often come across these patients when we treat with acupuncture.

When Liver yang is high and the yin weak (this is a serious imbalance in the Liver syndromes and is called Liver-fire or fire-heat in the Liver), there may be excessive and spontaneous bleeding from any organ or tissue.

Liver yin deficiency (Figure 3.19) can cause bleeding problems, and Liver Blood deficiency means there are problems with the Blood itself. These are both reasons for Blood deficiency in the body and dry, poorly nourished skin.

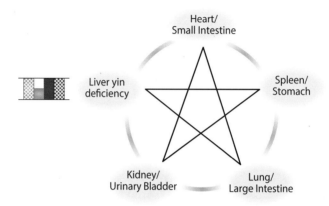

Figure 3.19 Liver yin deficiency

TABLE 3.3 COMPARISON BETWEEN LIVER YIN DEFICIENCY AND LIVER BLOOD DEFICIENCY

Liver yin deficiency	Liver Blood deficiency
Dryness – gritty eyes with recurrent conjunctivitis, burning, redness	Paleness – blurred vision, dizziness, light-headedness
Recurrent tendon inflammation contractures, poor extension, easy ruptures, poor healing, muscle pains worse in activity, muscle tension, difficulty to relax muscle tension, tendency for yang to rise – high blood pressure, spontaneous excessive bleeding (menstruation, epistaxis), delayed coagulation, tension, stress	Easily numbed arms and legs, improves with movement, weakness of muscles, poor endurance Tendency for wind symptoms – nervous itching, sneezing, wandering symptoms Sound and light irritability, sudden appearing symptoms, long menstrual cycles with scanty bleeding
Headaches during menstruation	Headaches after menstruation
Tense person – can be aggressive	Weak, nervous person – irritable

Dry, brittle nails, nail-bed inflammation	Bites nails, white patches on nails
Tongue sides cracked, red papillae	Tongue sides pale
Liver pulse deep and wiry	Liver pulse thin and hollow
Nervous tics and tremor, vomiting	Uncontrolled internal tremor, upward staring eyes, colic
Treatment	
Tonify Liver yin: Liv 5 (Luo) GB 40 (sedation), K 7 (often mother is dry too); water and salty foods are good; relaxation, meditation; Du 20, P 6; fish oils, cream, foods that are naturally sweet-sour	Tonify Blood: UB 17 (influential point), Sp 10 (sea of Blood), Ren 14, H 9, UB 15, SI 3 – tonify Heart yin and yang, GB 39 – influential point for bone marrow. Wind elimination points to eliminate Liver wind
Avoid sour foods, alcohol	

As Table 3.3 shows, Liver yin deficiency causes more nervousness, tension, aggression and heat symptoms, while Liver Blood deficiency manifests more dryness, weakness, poor endurance, irritability and cold symptoms. Both can give rise to wind symptoms.

Liver yin deficiency makes more wind-heat and Liver Blood deficiency makes more wind-cold. Liver Blood deficiency quite often causes wind symptoms, whereas Liver yin deficiency causes heat to rise – and this heat stirs the wind.

A common problem for patients requesting cosmetic acupuncture is deep wrinkles on the forehead and between the eyebrows. Botulinum (botox) injection is a short-term solution for these wrinkles, but this causes temporary paralysis of the muscles in this area and affects the sinuses.

We can treat these wrinkles reasonably well with acupuncture, or we can treat this area before the patient recovers from the effect of botox. But these wrinkles can return as surely as the patient returns for botox injections. We have to address the cause of the wrinkles particularly in this special area. Does the patient wrinkle up their forehead because they are tensed or stressed? Do they have a problem with seeing properly? Some patients are too vain to wear glasses, but have to tighten all the muscles around the eyes in order to see. Do they have a chronic allergic rhinitis or sinusitis that makes them tense up their facial muscles? As the forehead is also related to the Stomach, do they have a Stomach problem?

Not everyone who has stress is tense and nervous. Not everyone who is tense and nervous is suffering from excessive stress. It is the tolerance and attitude to stress that matters. In a Liver yang-dominant situation there is more muscle tension. But it is possible for the person to relax. The lower the Liver yin becomes, the longer it takes for the person to be able to relax. So those who are Liver yin deficient are nearly always tense and stressed regardless of how much work they have to do, and if they go on holiday it takes them a few days before they can begin to relax.

When a patient has body language indicating stress and tension we should address this at the same time as we treat the wrinkles. It is necessary to tonify the Liver yin, give some calming points, and treat the eyes or sinuses accordingly. In this way, the treatment of the wrinkles will be successful for a longer time.

POINTS TO TONIFY LIVER YIN AGAINST STRESS AND TENSION

- Liv 5, Lu 1, UB 13, Lu 7, P 6, Ren 14, UB 15 – the Front-mu and Back-Shu points of Heart and Lung are given in order to tonify the general energy state of the upper warmer, which is very successful in treating tension in the neck and face; these points are more useful on pale-faced rather than red-faced patients.

- Du 20, UB 62.

- Ex 2 (Tai yang), GB 14 for the eyes.

- Ex 1 (yin Tang), and LI 20 or St 3 and UB 2 for the nose and sinuses.

- GB 20 in both the above cases.

- Sp 10, UB 17 in allergic conditions.

- St 40 when there is excessive mucus.

- Iron supplement (I normally recommend Floradix – herbal iron formula).

- Ren 6, St 36, Sp 6 and Lu 9 can be taken to improve general energy.

- GB 34 can be used if muscles and tendons are very weak.

Liver Qi and Liver wind

Wind is a movement of Qi, which makes possible the flow of Blood, energy and fluid in the body. The free movement of Liver Blood is very important for the skin and all other tissues. This free flow is achieved by Liver Qi, which is also called wind.

Wind is often characterized as a pathogenic factor, but this is not strictly true. Wind is not always a pathogenic factor. Breeze would be a gentle version of wind, and this is necessary in creating movement in the Blood, fluid and energy in the body. Imagine 50 people in a room with closed windows. It would be very stuffy and everyone would want the windows and doors to be opened to enable the air to circulate. Many diseases, including skin diseases, improve in a seaside environment. Wind can therefore be therapeutic in removing energy blocks and stagnation in blood or fluid flow.

When it is not possible to have exterior wind to help us with this free flow, the Liver generates interior wind in order to keep this free flow. To keep the Blood, energy and fluid moving freely is a very important function indeed.

Liver Qi deficiency and Liver Qi stagnation

When the Liver Qi is deficient, there could appear many blocks in energy or Blood flow – such as 'globus' (foreign body in throat sensation), blocked emotions, constipation, localized oedema, varicose veins, blood stagnation causing muscle pain, dysmenorrhoea and even unequal muscle tension in the two sides of the body (Figure 3.20A).

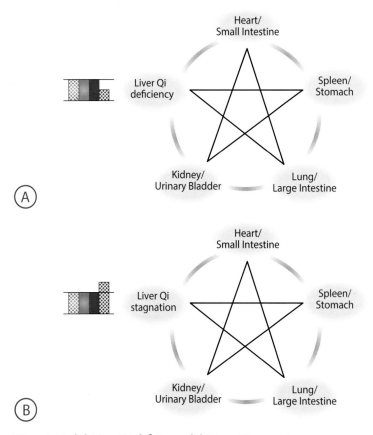

Figure 3.20 (A) Liver Qi deficiency; (B) Liver Qi stagnation

Liver Qi is generated in the interior through sports and harmonious exercises such as Tai Qi, Qi Gong and others. Also, slow stretching exercises such as Pilates are good. The Liver Qi especially helps with the venous blood flow; the Heart helps with the arterial blood flow; and the Spleen with capillary blood flow. Scientific evidence shows that people who are active and fidgety have fewer problems with their Heart and circulation. They certainly have more mobility and fewer locomotive problems. The Liver Qi is also important for the vessel tension and for maintaining good blood pressure.

The Liver Qi helps us to deal with anger in a healthy way. Those with a good Liver Qi can be assertive and reasonable, and at the same time convey their disagreement or dissatisfaction in a constructive way. Those who have a Liver Qi deficiency will bottle up their anger and become introverted and withdrawn while ruminating on their feelings. These bottled-up emotions will gradually build up and manifest as other symptoms such as hypertension, headaches, neurodermatitis, urticaria or bronchial asthma.

The diagnosis of Liver Qi stagnation is a very popular one. Every therapist makes this diagnosis when there are Liver symptoms that they are having difficulties diagnosing. The problems begin when our picture of imbalance is not clear as the treatment to balance it will then not be appropriate. These symptoms are demonstrated below.

This suppressed anger because of lack of power can manifest as hypertension, headaches, neurodermatitis, urticaria or tachycardia.

This can cause poor venous Blood flow and varicose veins or varicocele; also symptoms of Blood stagnation as clotty menstrual bleeding or Blood stagnation pains.

There can be a stagnation of cold and wet along the Liver meridian in the lower part of the body – manifesting in wetness, pain, numbness, genital itching, hydrocele and muscle cramps.

The first tower above resembles symptoms of Liver Qi stagnation, but is actually caused by Liver Qi deficiency. The following points will treat this situation effectively.

POINTS AGAINST LIVER QI STAGNATION CAUSED BY LIVER QI DEFICIENCY

- UB 18 – Back-Shu of Liver to improve its function.

- GB 37 – the Luo-connecting point, which will remove stagnation.

- LI 4 – the great eliminator, which will help eliminate blocked anger and frustration.

- St 40 – symptomatic point to circulate dampness.

Another representation of Liver Qi stagnation is shown below.

There can be an energy accumulation (not substance), as if suppressing expanding air into a container. Energy is blocked in the middle warmer – where the Liver is found. This may change into ascending wind or heat symptoms in the upper warmer, or manifest as fullness in the middle warmer or breast distension, as in premenstrual syndrome. Belching, with a feeling of upward pressure on the diaphragm, will also be a common symptom.

This is treated with heat or wind elimination, and points to cool, calm and eliminate excess in general.

- Local wind elimination points (pages 96–99) with the wind elimination sedation technique (page 105).

- Heat-elimination technique (page 102) on local points.

- Liv 3 – Yuan source point to harmonize the Liver.

- Liv 14 – Front-mu point to cool and calm the Liver.

- LI 4, St 25 – to eliminate fullness in the middle warmer.

- Sp 6 – ideally with descending technique (pages 105–106) to descend the ascending Qi.

- Ren 3 – also to bring focus to the lower warmer.

Excessive Liver wind

Liver wind can rise for many reasons:

- Liver Blood deficiency.

- Liver yang excess stirring wind-heat.

- Liver Qi stagnation.

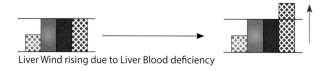

Liver Wind rising due to Liver Blood deficiency

This is a common cause of chronic fibromyalgia and chronic fatigue syndrome, particularly in women. Blood deficiency is more common in women than in men, because women lose Blood regularly through menstruation, and also through childbirth. They also tend to work around the clock, working at their job, running the home and looking after the children. There seem to be more demands on their energy and less rest and nutrition to fill their essence. As a result, the Blood becomes deficient and this can bring about a recurrent rising of wind.

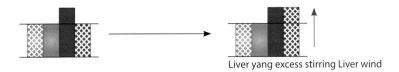

Liver yang excess stirring Liver wind

Liver yang can rise for many reasons – for example, anger, excessive alcohol or excessive irritation to the eyes through prolonged looking at a computer screen or colour television. When the yang rises, it will irritate the wind, causing wind-heat symptoms. These can include redness, itching or burning eyes and skin, neck tension and headaches and sneezing attacks with a blocked nose. The wind causes red blotchiness of the skin, irritability and wandering pains.

Liver Qi stagnation (both Liver Qi stagnation and Liver Qi deficiency)

These are two conditions with Liver Qi stagnation symptoms that I have previously described. In both conditions the Liver Qi rises from the middle to the upper warmer, causing pent-up emotions, extreme tension, headache, hypertension, urticaria and neurodermatitis. These are wind symptoms manifesting in the Liver and in other organs which are attacked by the Liver wind.

Wind symptoms may be:

- *Irritating* – itching, sneezing, irritation caused by light or sound, aversion to wind on skin and emotional irritability.

- *Wandering* – skin lesions or pain areas seem to wander around the body and are not fixed to one area.

- *Paroxysmal* – symptoms appear and disappear suddenly (allergic reactions, colicky pains and epileptic fits are examples).

- *Blocking* – a sudden wind symptom can cause an acute bi-syndrome (obstruction in a meridian flow, causing pain) or a wind stroke (one-sided paralysis).

Many skin diseases cause itching and have wandering lesions. We often see patients with more tension on one side of the face than the other and many patients have faces screwed up in pain but want to look pretty. Wherever possible, we should eliminate wind, disperse heat and alleviate pain. It is a tall order, and as long as we remember that we are treating the person as a whole and not just their face, we can fulfil our task reasonably well.

On page 64 I have explained why wind sometimes attacks the Heart and at other times the Lungs and the skin. I do not want to go into that again. What it is necessary to remember here is that wind is of a yang nature and even though it originates in the Liver it will attack wherever there is a yin or Blood deficiency. When the skin is attacked by wind, we should treat it by eliminating the wind from this area, and also by tonifying the Blood or yin, depending on which is deficient.

CASE STUDY

Let us consider a case of neurodermatitis in the face, neck and arms. The lesions are flat, reddish and wandering. The skin is dry and peeling; it feels tight like a mask. The itching worsens in heat and under bedcovers. The patient is restless and nervous and has problems with sleeping. The tongue shows some cracks at the centre and red papillae at the tip.

This is evidently a case of Lung yin deficiency with wind-heat on the skin. The nervousness seems to be from Liver yin deficiency and the Liver yang is making the wind rise and attack the Lung, which has a yin deficiency.

The treatment would be:

- Balance Liver – sedate GB 40 and tonify Liv 5 (tonify yin/sedate yang)

- GB 20, SI 12, UB 12 points with wind elimination sedation

- Tonify Lung yin with Lu 1, Lu 8, Ren 17 and perhaps K 10

- Wind elimination points and techniques are described on page 103.

CHAPTER 4

LUNG ASCENDS AND DESCENDS WATER

CHAPTER CONTENTS

This chapter is very short, and deals with the Lungs and the skin and their relationship with water. The chapter begins with a small diagram depicting water metabolism.

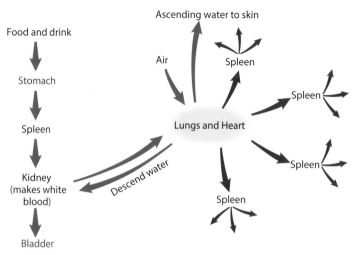

Figure 4.1 Lung ascends and descends water

Figure 4.1 shows how food and water are used to provide nutrition in the making of Blood; absorbed nutrition from the Spleen descends to the Kidneys, which also take part in Blood metabolism by making deoxygenated Blood in the bone marrow, and the Kidneys send the nutrition and the Blood to the Lungs. The Lungs and Heart oxygenate the Blood. This red blood is then circulated centrally by the Heart and peripherally by the Spleen to all organs and tissues of the body.

If the Heart yang is good but the Spleen yang is deficient, the body will be warm but the extremities will be cold. If the Spleen Qi is deficient, the hands and feet will receive less Blood and nutrition, resulting in dryness, numbness and poor wound healing.

The lungs are left with a residual amount of water after making the red blood, and have to get rid of the water – keeping just enough to moisturize the mucous membranes and the skin. The lungs send this water away in two directions:

- They *ascend the water* to the skin surface as sweat.

- They *descend the water* back to the kidneys to be stored or eliminated as the body requires.

Generally speaking, we sweat more (ascend) when hot and urinate more (descend) when cold, though both functions are continuous.

4.1   WHEN THE ASCENDING AND DISPERSING FUNCTION IS AFFECTED

A problem with the ascending function of the lungs principally results in skin problems.

First, the skin could be thick but dry with scaliness on the surface. This is because, even though there is dampness and fluid below the surface, the Lung Qi is deficient, and the skin pores do not open to disperse this fluid to the surface. The descending function may not be affected in this case, and there may not be any respiratory problems. Psoriasis and myxoedema are good examples of this imbalance.

TREATMENT TO HELP THE SKIN ASCEND WATER TO THE SURFACE

- UB 13 – Back-Shu point of Lung to improve function.

- LI 4 and LI 11 to help open the skin pores and disperse fluid to the surface.

- Hot and humid climate (or wet sauna/Turkish bath).

Second, the skin could be thin or hard, dry and rough on the surface, showing that there is less water in the Lung. This usually means that the Lung yin is deficient, and therefore the nose, throat and the mucous membranes will also be dry. This is not really a problem with the ascending function.

TREATMENT TO TONIFY LUNG YIN

- Lu 1, Lu 8.

- Ren 17, P 6.

- K 10.

- Drink more water.

- Inhale water vapour.

Third, the skin can be cold and sweaty. The sweat is very watery, and there is more sweat on the colder areas. The coldness is due to a yang deficiency on the part of the body which is cold. If the entire upper body and the arms are cold, this could also be a result of Heart Blood and yang deficiency.

Sweating when cold is caused by a defective Lung Qi, resulting in the skin pores being open and dispersing when they should be closed and keeping the heat and fluid inside.

Ascending and dispersing are functions but, more importantly, are necessary to correctly decide when the skin should disperse water and when the pores should close. This depends largely on the body temperature. The correct function of the skin is to maintain a constant body temperature.

> Failure of the skin to disperse fluid when the body is hot and sweating too much when the body is cold are both symptoms of Lung Qi deficiency.

TREATMENT AGAINST EXCESSIVE COLD SWEATING

- UB 13 and LI 11 – to improve Lung Qi.

- Lu 7 tonification and K 7 – to close the pores and stop sweating.

- UB 15, H 3 and SI 3 – to tonify Heart yang if the upper warmer is cold.

- Ren 14, UB 15, UB 17, Sp 10, GB 39 and iron supplement if the Heart is Blood deficient.

4.2 WHEN LUNGS DO NOT DESCEND WATER

Problems with the descending function can cause different symptoms. The descending function of the Lung does not concern us now, as this is a book on skin and beauty. Nevertheless, I would like to complete this picture of the Lung, as there is only this one opportunity to do so.

1. The lungs may be filled with phlegm. The phlegm is watery and foamy, not thick and gluey, and is easily expectorated. This causes coughing and asthmatic breathing, especially in wet and cold weather and at night and early in the morning.

There are two possible reasons for this. First, the Lung may have problems *descending the fluid* and therefore has excessive yin. Lung oedema would be a good example of this. It is therefore necessary to help the descending function of the Lung.

- Lu 5 sedation – Lu 5 is the water point of Lung and its sedation point. By sedating this point, we will be able to send the excess yin directly from the Lungs to the Kidneys.

- UB 13 and perhaps UB 17 with cupping – cupping therapy is helpful in removing fluid from the internal organs. The reason for adding more Back-Shu points is because the Lung is a large organ, and would benefit from more cups at the back of it.

- Use points K 24, K 25, K 26 and K 27. These last four points on the Kidney meridian are on the thorax, and are excellent for the descending function of the lungs.

2. The second reason could be that the Lung yin cannot descend into the Kidneys because *the Kidneys are full of yin and can receive no more water.* The symptoms of this can include oedema of the legs and reduced urine volume. In this case, the problem is with Kidney function, so we need to improve this in order for the the Kidney yin to return to normal and be able to receive the descending yin from the Lungs.

Points to improve the Kidney function to increase urine volume

- UB 23 – with needle and then cupping to improve Kidney function.

- UB 58 – Luo-connecting point of the Urinary Bladder to remove water retention.

- K 3 – the earth point and grandmother point of Kidney to increase yang.

3. There is a third way in which the Lung can be affected with phlegm. In this case, the phlegm is very *thick and gluey*, and the patient has problems with expectoration of this phlegm, whether from the nose, sinuses or bronchioles. The phlegm trickles down to the throat from the nose and sinuses causing catarrh, and the phlegm stagnates in the bronchioles and alveoli. This is, of course, due to Lung yin deficiency, the phlegm having insufficient thin fluid to circulate or expectorate it.

POINTS TO TONIFY LUNG YIN AND MAKE THE PHLEGM MORE WATERY

- Lu 1 – Front-mu point of Lung.

- Lu 8 – own-element point.

- Ren 17 – master point for respiratory system, given in the direction of the face.

- St 40 to improve circulation.

- K 10 – own-element point to improve general yin in body.

- Dry cupping on UB 13 and UB 17 to help expectoration in Lung problems; in neck and sinus problems, give cupping massage from hairline to scapula like a fan.

ADVICE FOR PATIENTS

- Drink water regularly, and take damp inhalation (add ginger to water to drink or inhale) in order to improve dispersion.

CHAPTER 5

ACUPUNCTURE POINTS, NEEDLE TECHNIQUES AND EXTRAORDINARY THERAPIES USED IN THE TREATMENT OF DERMATOLOGICAL AND COSMETIC PROBLEMS

CHAPTER CONTENTS

5.1 GENERAL TREATMENT POINTS

A. Du 20, P 6, An Mian points – for calming.

B. Liv 3, Liv 5 – against nervousness.

C. Sp 10, UB 17 – for cooling Blood-heat and purifying Blood, against pruritus.

D. Lu 5 sedation, Sp 9 – points to descend dampness (diuretic).

E. UB 13, LI 4 – points to disperse dampness (increase sweat).

F. UB 20, St 40, UB 39 – points to circulate dampness.

G. Sedation of LI 2, SI 8 and TW 10, needle UB 62 – points to disperse heat.

H. LI 4, St 25, TW 6 – points to improve elimination (against constipation).

I. Lu 1, K 10 and Sp 3 – points to improve nutrition and moisture to the skin.

J. Ren 17 – master point for respiratory organs, used also for the skin.

K. Wind elimination points.

GB 20 – for head and face.

UB 12 – for Lungs, back and skin.

SI 12 – for shoulder and arm.

GB 31 – for hip and leg.

Ba Xie – for hands.

Ba Feng – for feet.

The points listed above and shown in Figures 5.1 to 5.5 are generally used rather symptomatically, without much analysis. They are still very useful and employ different methods to disperse dampness from the three warmers; different ways to cool the body, dissimilar ways of elimination and for calming the person.

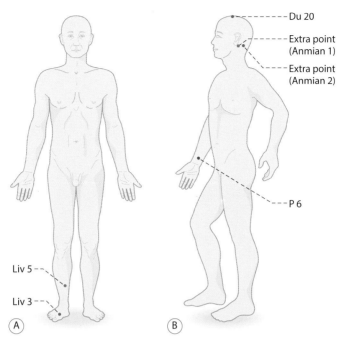

Figure 5.1 (A) Points against nervousness; (B) tranquillizing points

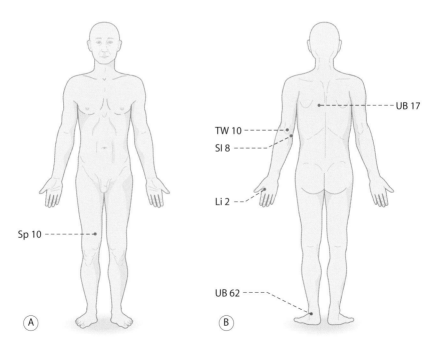

*Figure 5.2 (A) Points to purify and cool Blood-heat, calm pruritus;
(B) points to disperse heat, cool Blood-heat and calm itching*

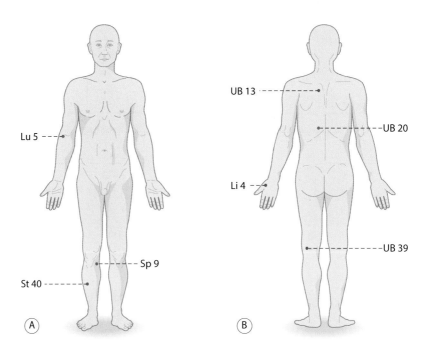

Figure 5.3 (A, B) Points to circulate, eliminate and disperse dampness

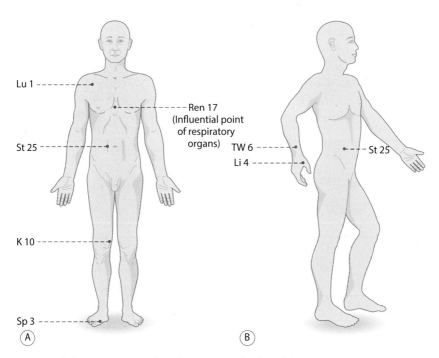

Figure 5.4 (A) Points to nourish and moisturize the skin; (B) points against constipation

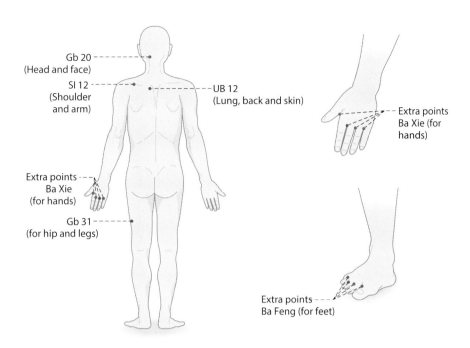

Figure 5.5 Wind eliminating points

For example, if the dampness is in the skin, points for dispersion [UB 13 and LI 4 (E)] and circulation (F) are often used. Points for descending [Lu 5, Sp 9 (D)] are used when there is dampness of the internal organ – the Lung.

The constipation points LI 4, St 25 and TW 6 (H) are used not only to regulate the stools, but also to improve elimination (of sebaceous secretions, of emotions, of menstruation) in general, and are great points to create a clear complexion.

Points Sp 10 and UB 17 (C) are used against allergies and itching. They are excellent points to cool heat in the Blood, and are also good for acne, carbuncles and folliculitis and other such surface inflammations of the skin. These are points that are used in almost every skin condition to purify the Blood and skin.

Points to disperse heat [LI 2, SI 8 and TW 10 sedation (G)] are mainly to sedate heat in the fire and metal elements, and UB 62 is the cardinal point of the Yang Motility (Yang Qiao) meridian, which cools the body.

Points Lu 1, K 10 and Sp 3 (I) are a combination of points to cool, nourish and moisturize the skin. When combined with regular drinking of water and nutritious food, these points can bring about a metamorphosis of the skin. If I were treating someone with thin and dry skin, I would use these points at each session.

Ren 17 (J) is the master point of the respiratory system. If we include the skin, we have three lungs. This point is important for skin problems. As this is a dangerous point and should be given subcutaneously, one has to decide which way the needle should point. If it points in the direction of the energy flow of the meridian, it will increase the yin of the skin and respiratory organs, and if it points against the direction of flow, it will reduce the yin in the skin and lungs (see Figures 5.1 to 5.4).

The wind elimination points are used against irritating symptoms such as itching, aversion to wind or cold on the skin. These points are invaluable in the treatment of allergic reactions – for example, sneezing, asthma, urticaria – and in all diseases with wandering or suddenly appearing symptoms such as headaches, rheumatism and skin lesions. Just needle the wind-eliminating point in the affected area and if you know it is a wind-heat symptom (most skin problems are), use the wind elimination sedation needle technique (see page 105); if it is a wind-cold symptom, then use the wind elimination tonification technique (see Figure 5.5).[1]

5.2　SPECIAL TREATMENT TECHNIQUES

- Sedation technique – to disperse energy.
- Dispersing fire technique – to disperse heat.
- Wind elimination sedation technique – to disperse wind-heat.
- Descending technique – to descend ascending heat.
- Bleeding technique – to expel heat or to remove Blood stagnation.
- Local needling – to improve local blood flow and circulation.
- Moxibustion – to warm and to dry wetness.
- Plum-blossom tapping – to increase yang on the skin or to release heat.
- Electrical stimulation of needles – to cool and disperse heat.
- Gua Sha – for treating small wrinkles and uneven skin (not scars).
- Laser – against inflammation and for cell regeneration and skin rejuvenation.

In addition to selecting general points against symptoms, other needle techniques and methods can be used to achieve various effects. Let us consider the above methods in detail.

1　The differential diagnosis of wind-cold and wind-heat and the relevant techniques are described on pages 103–105.

You may ask if it is necessary to perform so many different techniques to achieve the desired effect – is it not sufficient just to use some points on the body and many points on the face?

When treating a patient with Western medicine one would use a number of tablets, minerals, injections and beauty regimes, many of which have harmful side-effects and short-term cosmetic effect. With acupuncture, we must have points and needle techniques for what every tablet and injection is trying to achieve. To these techniques we add the energy-balancing treatment, which stabilizes the effect. And remember, we do not use all these techniques on one patient or in one treatment session. They are used in different patients and during different sessions. We should have the know-how if they are needed. Once you have learned these techniques and are using them regularly, they will become easy and you can work on autopilot.

Let us look at the techniques one by one.

5.2.1 Sedation technique

There are many sedation needle techniques that can be done. Sedation is performed to disperse energy away from the affected area, or from one meridian or organ. I mainly use two such techniques.

- *Needling against the direction of energy flow.* This method is used on a point that should be needled superficially – such as Lu 1, a dangerous point because of its proximity to the lungs, or Ren 17, GB 14 or Lu 7, which are all close to the bone and should be needled subcutaneously at an angle. You can have the needle pointing in the direction of meridian flow if you are tonifying and against the direction of flow if you wish to sedate.

- *Vibration technique.* The needle is first inserted into the point and needle sensation obtained. The needle is then held with as many fingers as possible, the hand is placed on the patient, and then the needle and the hand are vibrated continuously for between 30 seconds and 2 minutes, depending on how long the sedation should be applied. If it takes any longer, I would connect the needle to an electrical stimulator and stimulate it, in order to save labour.

The vibration technique could be done with a *much stronger twisting-twirling-lifting-thrusting combination,* instead of a light vibration. It is a question of whether the patient can tolerate such strong needling; after all, the purpose of sedation is to remove pain or excess energy and not to make the needling so painful that the patient feels nothing else.

Once the sedation technique has been applied, the needle can stay in the patient for 5–10 minutes in acute problems, and for 20–30 minutes in chronic problems. During this time, the sedation technique can be repeated, and repeated again shortly before removing the needle.

5.2.2 Dispersing heat technique

This is a simple and effective needle technique. Most importantly, it can be performed on any point, anywhere on the body, and it will only disperse heat. If the technique is performed on a sedation point (e.g. Liv 2) it might send the heat to the son organ, but if applied on a point such as Ren 12, it will actually disperse the heat outwards rather than to another organ. Therefore, it is a good point at which to disperse pathogenic heat.

The technique

Insert the needle at the point and obtain needle sensation. Then thrust the needle once (with one push) through the three levels of depth – heaven, man and earth – and lift three times, once through each level (Figure 5.6). One thrust, then three lifts – this is one circle of movement – repeat six times, the number for sedation. This creates coolness in the area in which you wish to remove heat. This technique can be used when dealing with acne rosacea, menopausal hot flushes, urticaria or eczema or even gastritis.

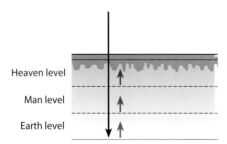

Heaven level

Man level

Earth level

Figure 5.6 Dispersing heat technique

This technique gives a similar result to that of bleeding. As it is not possible to apply the bleeding technique at all points of the body, this technique acts as a good substitute. The needle can be left for a minimum of 5 minutes, or 20–30 minutes when combined with other points.

5.2.3 Heat-introducing technique

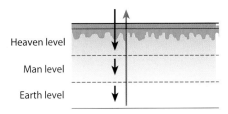

Heaven level

Man level

Earth level

Figure 5.7 Heat-introducing technique

This technique is the inverse of the dispersing heat technique. The yang is introduced from the exterior into the interior at three levels of depth. Again, this can be used on any point in the body, as the technique gives a clear message as to what should be achieved.

The technique

Insert the needle at the point and manipulate to achieve needle sensation. Then thrust the needle deeper in three movements (the total depth is decided by the thickness of muscle and fat in the corresponding area), and lift it to superficial level (not out of the skin) with one motion. Repeat this circle of movement nine times or more in nine sets (Figure 5.7). This should create a warm flow in the area of the needling. This technique is especially useful for those patients who cannot tolerate the smell of moxa.

This technique tonifies the yang of the area, meridian or organ – depending on the chosen point. For example:

- Using the heat-introducing method on the Front-mu or Back-Shu points will create more yang in the organ.

- Using it on the tonification point or fire point of a meridian would cause heat in the organ and meridian.

- Using the technique on a non-specific acupuncture point of an energy-balancing nature will only warm the area.

5.2.4 Wind elimination techniques

There are two wind elimination techniques:

- Wind elimination tonification technique (used in wind-cold).

- Wind elimination sedation technique (used in wind-heat).

Skin problems are more often caused by wind-heat, and therefore the sedation technique is frequently used. It is necessary, however, to be able to differentiate between hot and cold wind symptoms (Table 5.1) so that the correct technique can be used.

TABLE 5.1 COMPARISON BETWEEN WIND-COLD
SYMPTOMS AND WIND-HEAT SYMPTOMS

Wind-cold symptoms	Wind-heat symptoms
Skin looks pale or marbled, worse in cold weather; skin symptoms more constant	Skin looks red and feels hot; skin symptoms suddenly changing, severe
Affected skin feels cold, may have goosepimples, and patient feels better when skin is covered	Affected skin feels hot and worsens with heat, even though other areas of the body may be cold
Less thirst, preference for hot drinks	More thirst, preference for cool drinks
Urine and stools are lighter than usual for the patient	Urine and stool are darker than usual for the patient
Tongue has white coating	Tongue has yellow coating
Tongue body may be pale, especially on the sides	Tongue body may be red in specific areas
Pulse is wiry (wind character) and slow (cold)	Pulse is wiry and fast (heat)
Needs wind elimination tonification technique	Needs wind elimination sedation technique

The wind elimination technique is performed only on the wind-eliminating points (see page 99). The combination of the correct technique (Table 5.2) and the appropriate point will bring about nearly instantaneous results; similarly, if we diagnose incorrectly, and give the tonification technique when we should sedate or vice versa, the patient will instantly become worse.

TABLE 5.2 WIND ELIMINATION TECHNIQUES

Wind elimination tonification	Wind elimination sedation
Needle the wind-eliminating point, holding the needle as if needling both sides simultaneously, keeping the thumb in the lower position	Needle the wind-eliminating point, holding the needle as if needling both sides simultaneously, keeping the thumb in the lower position
Twirl thumb first towards centre, then away; repeat nine times	Twirl thumb first away from centre, then towards the centre; repeat six times
One lift and three thrusts (nine times)	One thrust and three lifts (six times)
Scrape handle towards body (nine times)	Scrape handle away from body (six times)
Leave needle for 5 minutes	Leave needle for 5 minutes
Remove during inhalation	Remove during exhalation
Close needle-hole	Leave needle-hole open

Other local, distal and energy-balancing points can be used simultaneously, while using the wind elimination point with the corresponding technique (Figure 5.8).

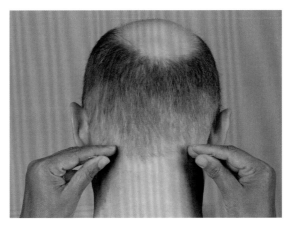

Figure 5.8 Correct placement of thumbs for wind elimination technique. Note direction of thumb-twirling for wind elimination sedation

5.2.5 Descending technique

This is a needle technique that is performed on only one point – Sp 6. It is used to bring down or descend the ascending heat from any part of the body to the lower warmer. This means that the heat symptoms are in the thorax, neck, arms and face, and markedly less in the lower part of the body. This technique is excellent for treating neurodermatitis in the upper body, or itching, heat rashes or allergic reactions manifesting only on the upper body.

> The Sp 6 descending technique can be performed up to three times in the first week of treatment; thereafter, it should be performed only once a week. It is contraindicated in patients with low blood pressure, bradycardia, angina pectoris and arrhythmia.

The technique

The patient should lie supine for this treatment, and no other needles should be in the patient at this time. The rest of the points can be needled later during the same session, or could have previously been in and removed.

- Needle Sp 6 bilaterally, just deep enough so the needles will stand at a right angle to the skin.

- Stands at the foot of the patient and cross your hands (your right hand against the patient's right leg, and left hand on left leg), and twirl the needle six times:.

  ○ In women – with the thumb, first up and then down.

  ○ In men – with the thumb, first down and then up.

- Then, tell the patient to inhale through the nose, swallow once (not to swallow air), and exhale through the nose. The patient should continue this breathing until you instruct them to stop.

- Push the needle in at Sp 6 as deep as you can without twirling. If you encounter the tibia, you should stop pushing any further.

- Repeat the twirling again at the deep level, and this time in both men and women twirl the needle with the thumb, first downwards and then upwards, six times.

- Perform three lifts and one thrust, repeating several times, with the needle becoming gradually more superficial (Figure 5.9).

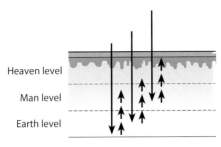

Figure 5.9 Descending technique

- When the needle has moved to a depth where it is just deep enough to stand without falling against the skin, leave the needle to stand for 1 minute. After 1 minute, you should prepare to remove the needle. Instruct the patient to change their breathing: keeping their hands on their Stomach, they should inhale through the nose and exhale heavily through the nose and mouth, and press the Stomach in while exhaling. The needle should be removed at the sixth exhalation.

- It is possible that the skin condition may move somewhat towards the skin in the lower body after a few descending treatments, but this will be a temporary phenomenon before the skin clears completely. Nevertheless, it is advisable to warn the patient of this possibility beforehand.

This might seem a difficult technique to master. You may have to refer to the book the first few times you perform it. Once you have done it a few times, try doing it without the book. You will soon be able to do it without a reference.

5.2.6 Bleeding techniques

Bleeding is used for two purposes:

- To eliminate heat.

- To remove stagnant Blood.

Eliminating heat

Heat is not always a bad factor. We need heat for warming, and in order to activate organ functions, the metabolism and functional Qi.

But heat can be a pathogenic factor. It can indicate the presence of an infection or inflammation – in which case it would inhibit the functional

Qi – and as such, this pathogenic heat should be eliminated and not transferred to another organ. Generally speaking, when the sedation point of a meridian is used in order to disperse excessive heat, this excessive heat will flow to the son organ – as the sedation point of a meridian is also the son point. But when a point is bled, this releases heat to the exterior. Sometimes, releasing only a few drops of blood will make an immense difference.

There are three techniques used to release Blood:

- Venous bleeding.

- Fingertip bleeding.

- Plum-blossom needle tapping.

Venous bleeding

This is used in order to create an effect on a large area – such as the entire upper body. It is ideal in the acute treatment of urticaria, acute skin inflammation on the upper body area, or even pneumonia or severe bronchitis.

CASE STUDY

I once treated a young woman (aged 28) with acute psoriasis. She had angry red patches of burning, itching skin involving her arms, neck, face and breasts – yes, breasts! It came on suddenly for the first time in her life when she had taken her two young children to visit her parents on holiday. The old couple felt unnerved by the active energy of the grandchildren, and she witnessed her father beating one of her children. She did not make a fuss about it at the time, but cut short her holiday and returned home. When she arrived home, the psoriasis broke out. It was so bad that she could not breastfeed her baby.

We treated her twice with Lu 5 venous bleeding and Lu 6 sedation, and she was much better within 3 days.

The case study above illustrates the unresolved anger creating wind-heat in the Liver and attacking the Lung and ascending to the upper warmer. With bleeding of the vein at point Lu 5, it was possible to eliminate heat from the Lung and the upper warmer.

THE TECHNIQUE

Using a hypodermic needle and syringe, draw out 3–5 ml blood from the vein, as close to the point as possible. Remove the needle and press to stop bleeding.

Fingertip bleeding

This treatment could be performed either on the finger- or toe-tips or on the jing-well points of the meridians. For instance, if the skin of the hand is very dry and the palm inflamed and itchy, the fingertips could be bled – especially at point P 9, as the meridian flows directly through the centre of the palm. The bleeding need only be done once or twice. This will release the heat in the hand, and when combined with needling of point P 8 to tonify yin, will make the skin soft and moist within three or four treatments (Figure 5.10).

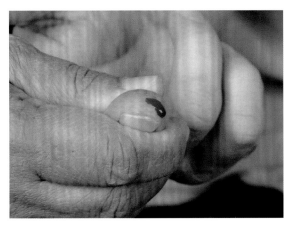

Figure 5.10 Fingertip bleeding

Fingertip bleeding is used to treat small joint inflammation, and is very useful in the treatment of psoriatic arthritis, for both conditions. The jing-well point bleeding is used more for releasing heat from the meridian and sensory organs – Lu 11 is bled in sinusitis or pharyngitis; St 45 is bled in herpes labialis.

When there is redness and itching/inflammation on the arm, maybe on the elbow fold, fingertip bleeding could be applied on the meridians that are affected. For instance, if the redness/eczema was along the ventral, medial side of the elbow, then the fingertips of the middle (Pericardium) and the small (Heart) fingers can be bled in order to drain the heat.

THE TECHNIQUE

Squeeze the finger around the distal phalangeal joint, and using a blood lancet or similar instrument make a quick puncture at the tip of the finger, and continue to squeeze and extract five to ten drops of blood. Apply pressure to stop bleeding.

Plum-blossom needle tapping

This is a very superficial bleeding technique, and is employed when removing heat in areas of thick and dry skin, or damp-heat situations. Flexural eczema with thick raised lesions would be a good candidate for this treatment. In this case, the cause of the skin condition is stagnation of dampness or blood. The heat appears because of the stagnant fluid. The dampness can be treated with points to circulate the stagnant fluid. But the heat needs to be eliminated from the surface. The plum-blossom hammer has seven short needles which, when tapped hard, will injure the epithelium of the skin and cause drops of blood to ooze. This will release the superficial heat on the skin and make the patient feel very comfortable afterwards. In fact, patients often itch themselves till they bleed, and this makes the irritation feel better.

THE TECHNIQUE

Hold the flexible handle of the plum-blossom needle and tap hard on the areas of the eczema several times, until blood appears on the skin surface.

Tap the entire area until it starts to show drops of blood. Stop tapping, wait one or two minutes, and then swab the blood (Figure 5.11).

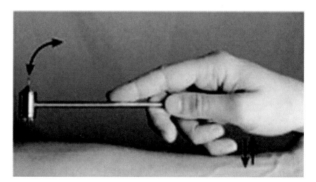

Figure 5.11 Plum-blossom tapping

It is good for the patient to take home their own plum-blossom needle, so they can use it when necessary. This treatment will create a noticeable change in the appearance of the skin the very next day – it will be flatter, pink and smooth instead of scaly, raised and rough. It will also make the pruritus better.

Removing stagnant Blood

In the treatment of musculoskeletal pains, this method is employed in the case of a deep-seated pricking or stabbing pain in a fixed area; in skin problems, this method is used mostly in treatment of varicose ulcers or varicose eczema. As the Blood return to the Heart is poor because of the varicose veins, there is Blood-heat and oedema in the legs. It is virtually impossible to improve the skin condition if the circulation does not improve. In such situations, Blood-letting is a quick and effective way to reduce the Blood-heat.

THE TECHNIQUE

The patient should sit or lie with a kidney tray positioned so blood will drip into it. Push in a hypodermic needle upwards into the vein, below a tortuous cluster of varicose veins, ideally distal to the varicose ulcer or eczema. Leave it there for 1 or 2 minutes to drip blood into the tray (Figure 5.12). Alternatively, one could draw blood out of the vein with a hypodermic syringe – about 3–5 ml.

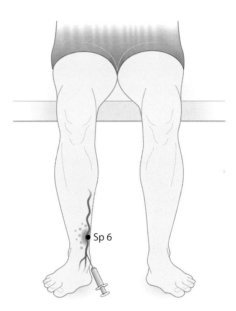

Figure 5.12 Venous bleeding below varicose ulcer

5.2.7 Local needling

We have often seen that the skin becomes red around the needled area. This shows that Blood and energy arrive at this area after needling. Local needling is a method that is employed to increase Blood circulation in areas where there is stagnation and Qi deficiency. It is excellent for use in acne vulgaris, cellulite and where wound healing is poor (Figure 5.13).

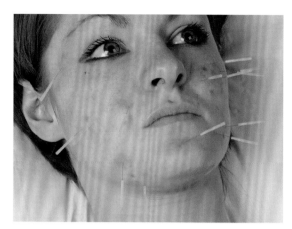

Figure 5.13 Local needling in acne. Needles are inserted superficially in the normal skin near acne pustules. Up to 15 needles can be placed in the face

The technique

Use 15-mm acupuncture needles of a 0.20-mm gauge.

- In patients with acne, insert around 15 needles superficially on the face. The needles should be applied near the acne, just deep enough to stand and not fall against the skin. They are left *in situ* for 20 minutes.

- In patients with cellulite, the same size needles are used, but the entire needle is inserted perpendicular to the skin. Approximately 10–15 needles should be used on each thigh and left for up to 30 minutes.

There is an immediate effect from these needles when they are extracted. The skin looks smoother and the affected area even feels lighter, and there is further improvement to be seen on the day after the treatment.

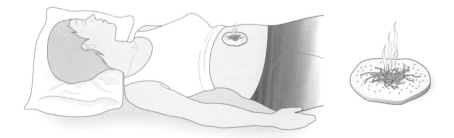

Figure 5.14 Ginger moxa

5.2.8 Moxibustion

The common moxa treatment for skin problems is ginger moxa. Moxa is a herb called mugwort, which is dried for 14 days in spring and then the leaves are crushed and burned like tobacco. Moxa is used on the skin – sometimes directly and sometimes indirectly with ginger or garlic in between.

Moxibustion is a heat treatment, and is generally used in cold, damp-cold or yang-deficient disorders. Warts, vitiligo and psoriasis of a cold nature are good indications for this treatment.

The technique

Cut fresh ginger into thin (1/8th cm) slices. Create holes in these with an acupuncture needle. Place the slices on the warts, vitiligo or psoriasis and thinly cover the slices with moxa wool. Light the moxa in several places and let it smoke. If the slices get too hot, hold the sides of the ginger plates and move them to another spot. Keep a saucer nearby in case the ginger slices become too hot in which case they should be thrown away.

If the affected areas are uneven and it is difficult to balance the smoking ginger plates, it is possible to cut fresh ginger and rub it on the affected skin, and then hold a lighted moxa cigar on this area. The addition of ginger to the moxa will make the effect more yang in nature. The ginger moxa has to be given regularly to the patient, daily if possible, and up to 14 treatments are required for best results (Figure 5.14).

Moxa is also used to increase yang in an organ. For instance, in the treatment of obesity, a moxa cigar is used on point Ren 12, in order to increase Stomach yang – to increase thirst and to reduce appetite – and is the most successful part of the treatment in promoting weight loss.

5.2.9 Plum-blossom tapping

The plum-blossom hammer has seven short, sharp needles grouped together on a flat surface. It can be used with a light tapping method to cause redness of the skin, or it can be tapped more heavily to cause bleeding.

Here we are referring to the light tapping method, which is effective in vitiligo for moving the Qi, and, more importantly, is used for firming the connective tissue on the chin, abdomen and anywhere there are fat tyres on the body, where the weight never seems to leave.

The technique

Hold the plum-blossom hammer at the handle and tap at a right angle to the skin along a line. The tapping has to follow a direction (these are described with the various therapy plans), and not in both upwards and downwards directions. The whole face of the hammer must fall flat on the skin with a 'thud' sound. Each hammered spot should be close to the earlier one, within 1 cm distance. You cannot hammer an 8 cm line in four taps. You will see a red line appear within 10 to 12 taps of a line. This will usually diffuse and widen within 1 or 2 minutes. Then you can move to tap the next one. Adjust the heaviness of the tapping if you see drops of blood appear – you are tapping too hard!

- For the treatment of *vitiligo*, one must tap daily till the depigmented skin is quite red. Each area needs 10 to 14 tapping sessions (and should be treated daily) before becoming pigmented.

- In lifting treatments to treat sagging face, arms, abdomen, etc. it would be sufficient for there to be one to two sessions per week to make a difference, and then once fortnightly or monthly for maintenance treatment.

- When treating 'tyres' (areas that stay fat and full, even though the rest of the body seems to become slim and supple), it is necessary to move the Qi in this particular area, so it will not stagnate and cause a block. To move the functional Qi, you can tap the paravertebral area behind this area vertically downwards on a line approximately 1 cm lateral on either side.

  - For 'tyres' on the chest area, the levels between C 6 and T 7 prominences can be tapped.

  - For 'tyres' on the upper abdomen, the levels between T 8 and L 2 can be tapped.

  - For 'tyres' around the lower abdomen and hips, the levels between L 4 and S 4 can be tapped (Figure 5.15).

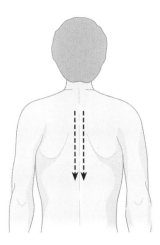

Figure 5.15 Plum-blossom tapping on lines 1 cm parallel to the midline. Lines are tapped downwards 10–15 times until a red skin reaction is obtained

In recent years, derma rollers have become popular. They have many more needles and can be of varying lengths and thicknesses. I don't think they make much of a difference, except perhaps they are easier for the therapist to handle. I feel that the most important practical tip is that plum-blossom tapping or derma rollers should be applied only in one direction, not both ways.

5.2.10 Cupping therapy

Cupping therapy is derived from an ancient therapy form using the horns of animals. Later, bamboo cups were used and then very elegant glass cups of various sizes and shapes. Cupping is basically a vacuum treatment and, though excellent in the treatment of musculoskeletal pains, it is very useful for a 'suction effect' on dampness in any form. In musculoskeletal pains, cupping therapy is best used for pains at the beginning of movement after rest. This pain takes 2–3 hours of activity following rest in order to improve, as this physical activity helps to create the Qi necessary for the dampness to be circulated.

In cosmetic acupuncture, cupping therapy can be used for the same reason – to help circulate stagnant dampness. The best results for this can be seen in the treatment of cellulite (see page 205). In this case, it is used as a massage aid. It is also excellent in oedema or lymph oedema treatment when used locally as retained cups or cupping massage.

The technique

There are many ways of administering cupping. The following ways could be used to attach the cup to the patient (Figure 5.16).

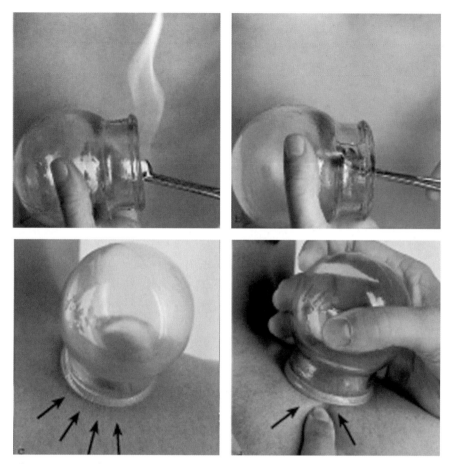

Figure 5.16 Cupping.

FIRE CUPPING

Attach to forceps a piece of cotton wool or gauze moistened with surgical spirit. Light the cotton wool and introduce it into the cup very quickly while still holding it with the forceps. This will create a vacuum in the cup by using up some of the air. Withdraw the burning cotton wool and place the cup very quickly onto the area to be treated. The greater the size of the fire and the quicker you transfer the cup, the greater the suction.

CUP WITH RUBBER PUMP

The rubber pumps on top of the cup should be squeezed before the cup is placed on the patient, and then released. This creates a vacuum, which sucks on the skin (Figure 5.17). These are more convenient for cupping massage, as one does not need fire to reinforce the vacuum each time to release it.

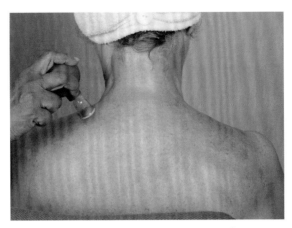

Figure 5.17 'Fan-like' cupping massage from hairline to scapula

CUP WITH MECHANICAL SUCTION

These are very new on the market. The cup comes with a suction gadget. Once the cup is placed on the patient, the suction can be regulated according to need.

MOVING CUP (CUPPING MASSAGE)

This can be done with ordinary cups or cups with rubber pumps.

Rub oil all over the area that is to be treated. If the intention is to create improvement in circulation, then a warming oil such as St John's wort oil, or any other oil that has been warmed prior to use would be suitable. Place just one cup at one end of the area using fire or suction, then run the cup along vertically, upwards and downwards – it is not necessary to go over the same line more than twice. The entire area should be covered with wide red lines (as wide as the mouth of the cup) when finished. This massage is quite painful if the cup is large and the suction is greater – it is easier for the patient if the cup is small and the suction is less. In treatment of severe dampness, such as cellulite, the suction should be greater to be more effective (see Figures 5.17, 5.18 and 7.12).

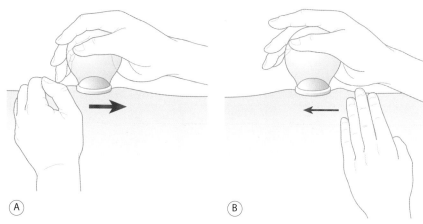

Figure 5.18 Cupping massage (moving cup)

When cups are retained *in situ*, it is sufficient to leave them on for 5–10 minutes.

5.2.11 Electrical stimulation of needles

Electrical needle stimulation is a newer addition to the established method from the 1960s. Its main use, in my opinion, is to reduce labour for the therapist. How so?

Manual stimulation of needles (1) is more painful for the patient, and (2) requires the therapist to stay by the side of the patient as long as the treatment is administered. If this manual manipulation is required for a longer time period, it is time-consuming and exhausting for the therapist. Moreover, if this has to be done on more than two points at a time, then the therapist would need more hands! For these reasons, it is so much simpler to have a machine to do this for you (Figure 5.19).

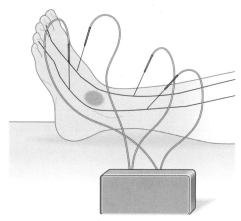

Figure 5.19 Electrical stimulation to disperse inflammation and itching

Electrical stimulation of needles can be used for achieving different results. In dermatology and cosmetic acupuncture, it is mainly used for cooling the skin, and for toning the muscles.

The technique for cooling the skin

Needles should be inserted above and below the areas where the skin is inflamed or hot. Needle handles should be connected to the clips of the same outlet in the electrical stimulator, and a continuous frequency of 5–10 Hz administered for 20 minutes.

For example:

- Sp 10 and Sp 9 for interior leg.

- LI 11 and Lu 6 for arms.

- UB 12 and UB 17 for upper back.

- UB 37 and UB 40 for upper leg.

- GB 30 and GB 31 for lateral leg.

- H 2 and SI 7 for inner arms.

CASE STUDY

A very young-looking female patient (aged 62) came to me complaining of pains in both feet and the coccyx for many years. Within the last 3 weeks she had developed a skin condition which was diagnosed as an urticaria. It started at the medial sides of both legs around the knees, and was now ascending to the inner thighs and to the fronts of her legs. When I saw her, the most recent areas were near point Sp 13 at the inguinal area. The patches were purplish, swollen and itchy and became a thick dry rash after a few days. The patient felt her clothes rubbing on the affected skin and this caused pain and some fluid to ooze from the area.

I felt she had some blood stagnation with heat, and treated her with points St 40 and GB 37 for the stagnation; and points Sp 10 and Sp 9 on both legs with electrical stimulation for the heat. She had only one treatment. Her symptoms subsided gradually within 4 days of the treatment.

Electrical stimulation of needles is contraindicated for patients with a pacemaker. Also, when attaching the clips from the electrical stimulator to the needle handles, it is important to keep the two clips from the same outlet on the same side of the body, and not cross sides, unless there is a special reason for doing so.

5.2.12 Gua Sha

Gua Sha is an ancient therapy associated with the extraordinary therapies of acupuncture. *Sha* means a disease caused by an attack of climatic pathogenic factors on the meridians, causing blocks and creating pain, coldness, stiffness or numbness of limbs and even fever or vomiting and diarrhoea. When the climatic factors attack the body for a period of time, they can also move to the interior, and affect the interior of the body in similar ways.

I am sure the reader has observed that on the exposed areas of the body the skin ages much more than the covered areas. So it is evident that the climatic elements take their toll on the skin and its associated tissues. The connective tissue forms an inner cover between the skin and the muscle, giving it protection and also firmness.

Facial Gua Sha

Facial Gua Sha is used slightly differently to body Gua Sha, which is mainly used to remove 'Sha' – the pathogenic factors that attack the body and need to be removed.

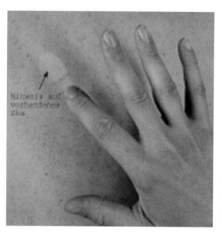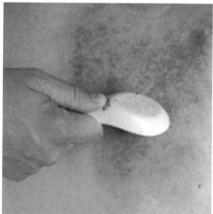

Figure 5.20 Gua Sha

With the various shaped Gua Sha instruments made with different materials, one could make wrinkles disappear, lift sagging jowls and hanging eyelids with immediate effect. And, with regular use, these changes remain and even improve.

Many a time, I have seen and heard audience gasp with wonder and disbelief after Gua Sha demonstrations on patients. The effects are excellent, especially on small wrinkles around the eyes and mouth, and the lifting effect it creates on brows, giving a 'wide-eyed look' and on the jaw line is extremely impressive. Gua Sha is given at a session where the patient lies down with constitutional points on the body for either thin and wrinkly skin (page 170) or against sagging puffy skin (page 182). No local needles are used on the face during this session.

Gua Sha sessions should ideally be given once per week, even though the temptation (because of the effect it creates) would be to treat more often. I also find that acupuncturist colleagues, who are somewhat wary of carrying out deep insertion of needles on the face, prefer to do only Gua Sha.

With Gua Sha treatment, we make many minute injuries on the superficial part of the skin at about the depth of the fine wrinkles, and this starts the healing process from within, where the skin would produce its own collagen to fill these wrinkles. While this healing process is taking place, it is better to leave the skin alone, without treating too often and causing disruption.

It is quite enough to do facial Gua Sha once per week and, every time to use the constitutional body points. But, if needed, the patient can be treated once more in the same week, when facial needles could be used against sagging or wrinkles.

The connective tissue

This is called the fascial connective tissue. According to Arya Nielsen (1995)[2]:

> The top layer of the superficial fascia is the fatty layer which acts as an insulator, helping to maintain a constant body temperature. Adipose tissue is metabolically active: it stores fat as fuel for metabolic function and releases it in response to nervous and hormonal stimuli. This corresponds to the Eastern concept of the greasy layer where the ancient Chinese Wei or Protective Qi circulates.

> The deep layer of superficial fascia lies immediately over the deep fascia and is less dense than the deep fascia. Arteries, veins, nerves, lymph vessels and nodes run through this bottom layer of the superficial fascia rather than between the layers. These vessels become surrounded by the fascia they penetrate and are thereby connected and held in place.

---

2   Arya Nielsen, *Gua Sha: A Traditional Technique for Modern Practice.* Oxford: Churchill Livingstone, 1995, p. 23–25.

Just below and adherent to the superficial fascia is the deep fascia. It covers most of the muscles, all the large blood vessels, all the large nerves, the deep lymphatics and nodes and certain glands.

On meeting any of these structures, the deep fascia splits into laminae, which surround the structures then reunite. A layer of this fascia can also split into many layers to enclose a space. There is not a cell or space that the connective tissue does not integrate.

The fibrils of connective tissue have a degree of crystallinity; the alternative compression and expansion of the crystalline lattice creates a piezoelectric effect. Voluntary muscular movement, even the continuous activity of cell motion, leads to the compression necessary for electrical field generation. Oschman (1987)[3] demonstrates that these fields expand through the tissues, producing signals that alert the cells. In response, the cells use this information to alter their actions of nourishing and maintaining the surrounding tissue.

Heat and movement keep the ground substance fluid, facilitating transit and conduction. Disuse and subsequent lack of warmth can cause the fluid ground substance to gel and the collagen fibrils to bunch and glue. This results in thickening and shortening of the connective tissue, which may even bond to its underlying tissue, creating adhesions. The end result is constriction of movement, slowing of metabolic processes and compromised immunity.

> Movement and stretching breathe life into connective tissue. Pressure, friction, massage and acupuncture, as well as other tactile stimulation, create fascial events. Piezoelectric signals stimulate chemical changes which signal cells. Gelling ground substance fluid warms, loosens and liquefies, which increases conductivity and metabolic transit. Static, excess fluid is astringed. Febril gluing and resulting adhesional constriction is discouraged. The immune function of connective tissue is quickened.[4]

The connective tissue is mainly nourished by Spleen Blood and is given continued firmness by Spleen Qi. To fully utilize the nutrition and fluid and to improve the Qi and firmness, tactile stimulation of the connective tissue is obviously of the foremost importance. This is the reason that the Gua Sha technique is being used here.

---

3   James L. Oschman, *The Connective Tissue and Myofascial Systems.* Berkeley, CA: Aspen Research Institute, 1987.

4   Nielsen (1995), p. 23–25.

Through the use of the Gua Sha technique, I try to reinvigorate the connective tissue – especially on the areas of the face and neck that are ageing and badly wrinkled because they are exposed to the elements – to rejuvenate these areas, nourishing and maintaining them, warming them and improving suppleness and activating the fibroblasts resulting in more ground substance and collagen production.

A sagging face lifted with needling produces good results. But the small wrinkles around the eyes, the mouth, on the neck and décolletage are very difficult to change. With the Gua Sha technique there is a marked improvement, especially in the long term. The disadvantages of this treatment are that (1) there is some redness noticeable for a day or two after the treatment (this can easily be removed with jade rollers and cooling creams applied at the end of treatment), and (2) it requires a longer time with the therapist at the patient's side to administer the treatment – this means that the therapist can only attend to one patient at a time.

THE TECHNIQUE

The technique is described in detail on page 173.

Gua Sha treatment is performed:

- Once a week for the first four sessions.

- Once in 2 weeks for a further two sessions.

- Once a month, but only if necessary.

The patient should avoid direct sunlight until the redness subsides, or the skin could become hyperpigmented, especially if St John's wort oil has been used.

Unlike Gua Sha carried out for musculoskeletal problems, the strokes are always in the upwards and outwards directions, as shown in Figure 5.21.

5.2.13 Laser

The most recent addition to cosmetic acupuncture, laser used together with needling, creates superb results. With laser, we can achieve deeper penetration and greater cell rejuvenation with soft and painless therapy. It is also extremely effective in the treatment of skin diseases such as eczema, acne, varicose ulcers, and so on. The therapy times are short and patients are pleased with the results.

There are special cosmetic laser applications nowadays that have specific frequencies for treating various problems. The techniques are simple: some starter information is needed, but then is they are very easy to follow. The most recent innovation, the Polylaser Derma, alpha frequency, used with hyaluronic acid for skin rejuvenation, is an excellent addition to cosmetic acupuncture. It gives the final touches for fine wrinkles and unclean-looking skin – leaving the skin smooth, glowing and radiant. Hyaluronic acid, which is massaged into the skin and not injected, penetrates deeper when the skin is warmed to open the pores. The laser actually promotes cell rejuvenation. The combination of these two therapies, if the therapists can afford them, will not only slow down the ageing process, but also erase and prevent fine lines.

CHAPTER 6

COMMON DERMATOLOGICAL DISEASES
Their Analysis and Therapy

CHAPTER CONTENTS

In this chapter, I wish to talk about some of the dermatological diseases in which acupuncture treatment has given good results. In each case, I will give a short summary of the general symptoms and treatment (for the reader's quick reference), and then go on to explain further. In some cases, I have included the Western viewpoint as a parallel.

I have described two main types of neurodermatitis below. There could, of course, be mixed types or other uncommon types.

I have to say at this point that, as a rule, all skin problems relate to the Lung. But they do not appear over all the skin, only in certain areas in each patient. This is because the meridian along which the disease manifests plays a role. Sometimes it is only a problem of the meridian, and it is sufficient to balance the meridian for treatment, and give only point *Ren 17* as a master point for skin and Lung. This is a rule that could be used for all skin disorders and musculoskeletal pains.

6.1 NEURODERMATITIS AND ECZEMA

6.1.1 Wind-heat in the Lung

The following types of illness can be compared with the wind-heat symptoms in traditional Chinese medicine (Figure 6.1).

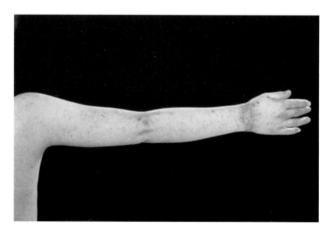

Figure 6.1 Neurodermatitis

Atopic dermatitis is one of the most widespread and worrying forms of eczema. Atopy means an inherited state of hypersensitivity, which may manifest itself as asthma, hay fever or eczema. It is more common in earlier life, occurring at some stage during childhood in up to 10–20 per cent of all children. It is a genetically complex, familial disease with a strong maternal influence.

The disease is also significantly influenced by environmental factors.

Infection either in the skin or system can lead to an exacerbation, possibly by a superantigen effect. Strong detergents, chemicals and even woollen clothes can be irritants and exacerbate eczema. Teething is another factor in young children. Severe anxiety or stress is a very strong factor in irritating the skin. Cat and dog fur can certainly make eczema worse, possibly by both allergic and irritant mechanisms. Food allergens could play a role in triggering atopic eczema and dairy products may exacerbate eczema in some infants.

Senile or winter eczema is dry, cracked skin with red erythema. It occurs more in the elderly, and predominantly in the lower legs and hands, especially in winter.

Lichen simplex/neurodermatitis. Lichen is a term applied to a group of chronic skin diseases characterized by thickening and hardening of the skin, with the formation of papules. Lichen simplex develops as a result of persistent scratching. The disease is more common in women than men. In women, it occurs most commonly in the nape of the neck, the back of the forearm, the inner part of the thigh, the back of the knee and around the ankles. The skin becomes thickened and has been likened in appearance to Moroccan leather.

This wind-heat type is very common in the West. It manifests as itchy erythematous scaly patches without clear edges, especially in the flexures such as the front of the elbows, behind the knees and around the neck. In infants, it often starts in the face before spreading to the rest of the body. Scratching may produce excoriations, and repeated scratching produces skin thickening with exaggerated skin markings.

In dark-skinned patients, there could be hyper- or hypopigmentation of the inflamed areas, which may change very slowly.

TABLE **6.1** NEURODERMATITIS – TRADITIONAL CHINESE MEDICINE VIEW

Wind–heat in Lung	Treatment
Thin, dry skin, less body hair, wandering flat, dry lesions without clear edges	Tranquillizing: Du 20, Liv 3
	Cooling Blood-heat: Sp 10, UB 17. Thin and dry skin: K 10, Sp 3. Wind-eliminating points with sedation
Skin appearance and itching worse with alcohol, sour food, stress and hot weather	
	Energy balance: Lu 1, Lu 8, Ren 17 in direction of flow; sedate SI 8, TW 10 and GB 38; bleeding finger-/toe-tip or venous bleeding on Lu 5; no alcohol or citrus fruits; avoid pickled or sour foods
Nervous person, emotionally up and down	
Can suffer from hay fever and allergic asthma	
	Two sessions per week for 3–4 weeks; one session per week for 4–6 weeks; one session every 2 weeks for 2 months; one session per month for 6 months
Better during pregnancy and humid, cool weather	
Hard stools, may be abdominal colic	

When treated aggressively with steroid creams or oral steroids, the skin actually becomes dryer and flakier. If this neurodermatitis is suppressed, it could move to the interior and cause asthma. The best way to approach balancing is to improve the yin and Blood, and this should calm the wind-heat. This is the worse of the two types, covering large areas of skin and causing more itching and irritation to the patient – but this is also the type that responds dramatically to acupuncture!

Explaining the treatment

For tonifying the yin of the skin and Lung, points Lu 1 (Front-mu point) and Lu 8 (metal point or own-element point) are used. Point Ren 17 is the master point of the respiratory organs and also the skin. The skin is said to be our third Lung. When Ren 17 is needed for increasing Lung yin, it should be given in the direction of the meridian flow.

Another point that is very effective in increasing the yin of the skin is point K 10, the water point or the own-element point. This tonifies the yin in the Kidneys so that they can irrigate the entire body, and point K 10 draws yang away from the large intestine, from the opposite side of the organ clock. This, in turn, reduces the Lung yang indirectly, as it is the coupled yang organ to the Lung.

A combination of points Lu 1, K 10 and Sp 3 have been mentioned before as a good prescription against thin and dry skin, and all these points are found in this treatment plan. Lung (and skin) gets its yin from the Kidney and its nutrition (Blood) from the Spleen. It is for this reason that point Sp 3, the earth point and the own-element point, is used.

The own-element points are used here to tonify the house energy of the organs – point Sp 3 tonifies Spleen yin/Blood; Lu 8 tonifies Lung yin; and K 10 tonifies Kidney yin, as these are all yin organs.

Advice for patients

Patients should improve their nutrition by including in their diet some proteins (taking care to avoid meats and fish to which they might be allergic), milk or buttermilk, some oil in marinating foods and in salads and rice (as white rice improves Lung Blood) – this treatment would work very well.

6.1.2 Damp-heat in the Lung

There are quite a few differences between wind-heat and damp-heat type eczema. If in doubt about the damp and yin situation in the skin (because that is the basic difference), one can perform a simple test of dermographia on the skin. The test is best done on the ventral side of the forearm. Scratch a long, firm line on the arm with your nail or a blunt instrument. In an allergic person this leaves a raised, red mark. But if the Lung/skin had less yin and Blood, this would leave an unraised white mark.

This second type of eczema is of a typically yin nature, as it stays in a fixed locus and does not change very much. Because the skin changes in structure in the affected areas and because it is often on the nape of the neck, popliteal, inguinal and cubital folds, the skin can crack and bleed and be quite painful. Healing is not quick and clothes can stick to the oozing body fluids from the lesions and it hurts to move.

The following three conditions fit the damp-heat in the Lung skin description.

WESTERN MEDICAL CONCEPT

Seborrhoeic dermatitis can present as 'cradle cap' in infants; a more widespread erythematous, scaly rash can be seen over the trunk, especially affecting the nappy area.

In young adults, there could be erythematous scaling along the sides of the nose, in the eyebrows, around the eyes and extending to the scalp, which could show dandruff.

Discoid eczema is a morphological variation of eczema, characterized by well-demarcated scaly patches especially on the limbs, and this can be confused sometimes with psoriasis. It is more common in adults and can occur in both topic and non-topic individuals. It tends to follow an acute/subacute course rather than a chronic pattern. There is often an infective component.

Varicose eczema occurs on the lower legs because of chronic venous hypertension (usually of more than 2 years' duration). The exact cause remains unknown but it has been suggested that venous hypertension causes endothelial hyperplasia and extravasation of red and white blood cells, which in turn causes inflammation, purpura and pigmentation.

Explaining the treatment

Unfortunately, true to its yin nature, this type of eczema does not respond quickly to acupuncture. The treatment is directed towards circulating and eliminating dampness. Even though the patient is not particularly constipated, the constipation points – St 25, TW 6 and LI 4 – are used along with Sp 9 for diuresis and St 40 for circulating fluid. These points will reduce the quantity of thick fluids the skin has to deal with.

Points UB 13 and LI 4 also help the skin function of dispersing fluid to the skin surface. Lu 5 descends fluid to the kidneys, thus reducing the stagnation of fluid.

The heat emanates from the stagnant dampness, and will disappear on its own accord if the dampness is removed. However, some superficial treatment for removing heat can be used, and this is plum-blossom tapping on the lesions. The tapping is carried on until there are droplets of blood on the itching areas, and the blood is wiped off. This will lead to an improvement in the appearance of the lesions on the very next day after treatment. The areas will look red (not purple) and be much smoother and softer. The patient could take the plum-blossom hammer home, and use it when she feels the need to scratch.

TABLE 6.2 ECZEMA – TRADITIONAL CHINESE MEDICINE VIEW

Damp-heat in Lung	Treatment
Thickened, scaly and hyperpigmented areas of lichenification. It starts with intense itching that becomes tender with increased itching and rubbing. Worse in wet weather, with damp-producing foods	General points: Du 20, Liv 3. Against Blood-heat and pruritus: Sp 10, UB 17
Becomes worse during pregnancy and before menstruation. Dairy products and wet weather also aggravate it. Melancholic person	Energy balance: LI 4, TW 6, St 25 – for elimination; St 40, Sp 9 – against dampness; Lu 5, UB 13 – to descend dampness and improve skin function
Can suffer with blocked nose or yin asthma	Plum-blossom tapping to bleed on affected areas
Stools tend to be semi-solid	Avoid dairy products and refined sugars and carbohydrates, and cold and raw foods
	One session per week for 8 weeks; one session every 2 weeks for 3 months; can start a fresh course after 1–2 months' break if improvement is good

SUGGESTIONS FOR LOCAL TREATMENT FOR BOTH TYPES OF DERMATITIS

- Dry and itchy palms – point P 8 needled only.

- Dry and itchy soles – point K 4 with heat-eliminating technique.

- Dry and itchy knee-fold – points K 10 and UB 40, needled.

- Dry and itchy elbow-fold – Lu 5 with heat-elimination technique.

- A red itchy lesion with clear edges on a meridian – place two needles on the meridian, one above and one below the lesion. If there are two meridians flowing through, then unblock both (Figure 6.2).

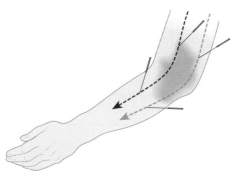

Figure 6.2 Local treatment of eczema

6.2 ACNE

I discuss three types of acne below. I have described the acne as I see it, and the analysis and treatment are carried out according to these symptoms. Again, there may be several more manifestations of acne and many mixed types.

6.2.1 Acne vulgaris

> **PATHOPHYSIOLOGY OF ACNE – A WESTERN MEDICAL CONCEPT**
>
> - Increased production of sebum, manifested as greasy skin.
> - Proliferation of commensal bacteria, in part connected with increased production of sebum.
> - Blockage of the follicular opening due to hyperkeratosis of epithelium in the follicular canal, which is the basis for comedone formation.
> - An inflammatory reaction to commensal bacteria and hyperkeratosis.
> - In women, increased androgen values may be relevant, especially in association with polycystic ovary disease.

Acne vulgaris manifests as large deep-red pimples with yellow heads. It affects predominantly the face but also the neck, décolletage and upper back. The pimples become darker after the pustules heal and form deep scars which remain, making the skin seem quite uneven. Post-inflammatory scarring, keloid scarring and pigmentation can last for over a year. The condition is common in teenagers and is often worsened by their diet of refined sugars and milk products, but it is also seen in adults (Figure 6.3).

> ## TRADITIONAL CHINESE MEDICINE VIEW
>
> - Poor elimination of skin – Lung (and LI) Qi deficiency.
> - Deep scars that remain after healing, making skin very uneven – signifies yin deficiency and the fluid being too thick.
> - Thick oily skin – dampness in Lung (and Spleen).

Treatment

- Reduce dampness – Lu 5 sedation (perhaps also Sp 9).

- Improve circulation – UB 13, St 40, many local needles.

- Promote elimination – LI 4, St 25, TW 6.

- Cool the heat – Sp 10 or UB 17.

- Disperse heat – Lu 5 venous bleeding.

- Avoid dairy products and refined sugars to counter dampness.

- Treat twice weekly for 12 sessions.

- The highlight of the treatment is the local points on the areas of the acne.

THE TECHNIQUE

I use 15 mm needles of a 0.20-mm gauge for this. With the patient lying down, place many short needles subcutaneously at the areas where the acne is prevalent. The needles should be given just deep enough to stand, and not fall against the skin. The needles are given in the normal skin, not in the inflamed area. There can be up to 15 needles on the face. Leave the needles for 20 minutes, along with the other acupuncture points on the body. No needle technique is used and no De Qi is obtained. This local needling causes the maximum effect on the acne, where the skin clears after each treatment. The patients love the effect, and never complain about the pain. The results are due to the fact that the local needling causes increased blood flow and circulation in the area.

The primary problem in acne vulgaris is the thick and oily skin and an increased sebum production from the sebaceous glands. This is worsened by a poor diet, which is very damp-producing – refined sugars, milk products, oily foods and eating large meals in the evenings. The dampness originates in the Spleen, and affects the lungs and skin. The points Sp 9 and St 40 will help this. Patients should be given strict instructions on what to avoid in their diet. If they follow the advice when treatment begins, they will see a great improvement, and this will keep them motivated. If at any time they return to their poor eating habits, they will see the skin immediately worsen. Often, patients ask us how long the effects of the treatment will remain. We can tell them that it will be good for as long as they take care of their diet!

There are many of us who have oily skin but without acne. Problems begin when the skin does not eliminate the sebaceous secretions well, and these stay under the skin and create stagnation of dampness. There could be two reasons for the problem:

- The Lung Qi is deficient, and the skin has poor opening and eliminating functions, so the dampness cannot get out.

- The thick fluid of the sebaceous secretion has less thin fluid – yin deficiency – and therefore the fluid becomes even thicker and this makes the circulation and elimination of the fluid more difficult. This also affects the healing process, and the scars remain deep long after the pustules have healed.

The treatment for the first problem is to improve elimination. It is interesting to note that many patients with poor elimination of the skin also have problems with constipation. Treat the constipation, and the skin improves its elimination function. Hence the points LI 4 (the great eliminator), St 25 and TW 6 are used. Also, tapping with the plum-blossom hammer along the para-vertebral line from the level of L 4 to S 4 until there is a red skin reaction will help with activating the bowels. For the skin itself, points UB 13 and LI 11 will help to activate the Qi.

ADVICE FOR PATIENTS

Good skin hygiene is crucial in the treatment of acne. Many patients use extra make-up to cover the acne but do not remove it thoroughly. This blocks the pores and worsens the situation. We should advise patients to clean and steam the face morning and night, and to use a light moisturizer afterwards. A facial sauna is also a good idea.

The treatment for the second problem is to tonify the yin. Patients should drink water (ideally warm) throughout the day. This will thin out the thick damp fluid of the sebaceous secretions, and improve its circulation and elimination movement. Point Lu 1 will also help to thin the sebaceous secretions.

Cooling the heat or treatment of the inflammation is done with point Sp 10 or with UB 17, both of which are excellent points against any surface irritation or inflammation. However, if a large area of the skin is affected, venous bleeding on point Lu 5 can be used once or twice.

Take note: many patients with acne vulgaris take long-term oral antibiotic treatment. The skin flares up very badly when they stop this for the acupuncture treatment. Unfortunately, these patients are not good subjects for acupuncture as we seem to be working on them at the worst possible moment. We would be wasting the precious first few treatments on them, as their bodies are likely to have a poor response. It would be best if they stopped taking the antibiotic, waited a month, and then came for treatment. They could use topical creams during this time to ease the symptoms.

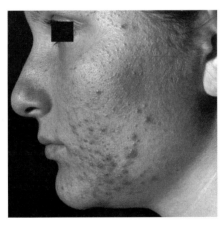 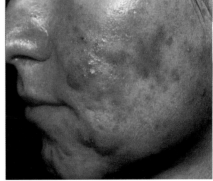

A   B

Figure 6.3 Acne vulgaris

6.2.2 Acne rosacea

ACNE ROSACEA – TRADITIONAL CHINESE MEDICINE VIEW

- Rather pale skin – Lung yin deficiency (Heart Blood deficiency).
- Sudden appearance of flushed areas on face, with burning or irritation – ascending Lung yang.
- Symptoms appear suddenly with alcohol, heat or anxiety – wind.
- Can become more permanent red erythema in later stages – heat.

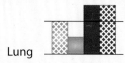

Lung

TREATMENT

- Local points only around pustules as in acne vulgaris.

- Tonify Lung yin – Lu 1, Lu 7, Ren 17.

- Tonify Kidney yin – K 10, water.

- Descend the ascending heat – Sp 6 descending technique.

- Eliminate wind-heat – GB 20 wind elimination sedation technique.

- Two sessions in the first week, followed by one session weekly for 4 weeks, then one session every 10 to 14 days depending on the improvement. If the patient is very pale, the Heart Blood should also be tonified.

It is quite common for patients with acne rosacea to have a pale complexion, especially in the early years of the disease, but this is not always the case. In patients who are pale, it is necessary to rule out symptoms of Liver or Heart Blood deficiency. This is because it is a wind symptom, and wind occurs more often in the case of Blood deficiency than yin deficiency. If the patient complains of easily sleeping extremities that improve with movement, blurred vision, scanty menstrual bleeding with long cycles, weak muscles and tired eyes, these could be signs of Liver Blood deficiency; if she has symptoms such as poor concentration and memory, poor sleep, feeling hot or cold easily with cold sweating, a weak voice and endogenous depression, this could be Heart Blood deficiency. In both cases, the following points would be useful: Ren 14, UB 15, Sp 10, UB 17, GB 39, Liv 8 and P 6. The patient could also be recommended a herbal syrup with iron or an iron supplement.

If the patient has no symptoms of Blood deficiency, this part of the treatment can be omitted.

As acne rosacea is a wind-heat disease symptom, it is necessary to eliminate wind-heat directly from the area it manifests. Hence the *wind elimination sedation* of point GB 20 (see pages 103-105).

Since the wind-heat appears on the skin and on the face, there must be a deficiency of the yin aspect of the Lung. If not, the wind-heat will not affect the Lung – it will affect another organ that has a weakness. In order to tonify Lung yin, points Lu 1 and Lu 7 are used. Lu 1, the Front-mu point of the Lung, has the function of cooling it, and Lu 7, the Luo-connecting point, not only *tonifies the yin* but also *sedates the yang* of the Large Intestine and the Lung. Point *Ren 17*, the master point for the respiratory organs and the skin, is needled in the direction of energy flow of the Ren meridian, in order to tonify the yin. These three points tonify Lung yin, sedate Lung yang and prevent the wind-heat from affecting the Lung and skin.

The wind-heat here appears in the upper part of the body, and we call it an ascending symptom. It is therefore important to descend the wind-heat. This is achieved by Sp 6 (the area distal point for the lower warmer) *descending technique* (see page 105). This, together with tonifying the Kidney yin, will bring more yin to the lower warmer, and stop the wind-heat ascending to the upper warmer. Sp 6 descending technique is used very successfully in post-menopausal hot flushes along with Kidney yin tonification. It would help immensely if the patient drinks water throughout the day and avoids excessive coffee or alcohol.

DIFFERENCES BETWEEN ACNE
VULGARIS AND ACNE ROSACEA

Acne vulgaris

- Peak prevalence is between middle and late teenage years.
- Papules, pustules, comedones (blackheads or whiteheads) and nodules.
- Scarring.
- Improves with sunshine.
- Can affect chest and back.

Acne rosacea

- Peak prevalence in patients aged between 40 and 70.
- Facial flushing, burning, later papules, pustules and blepharitis.
- Soft tissue overgrowth in the form of rhinophyma.
- May worsen with sunshine.
- Usually limited to the face.

During the later years of acne rosacea, the skin erythema becomes permanent. Dilated blood vessels, inflammation of the eyelid margins (blepharitis), keratitis and sebaceous gland hypertrophy, especially of the nose, appear. The treatment is still the same, except some adjacent points around these areas can be included.

6.2.3 Prickly heat

I call this acne 'prickly heat', for want of a better description, as it looks more like a heat rash. The papules are small and have sharp red heads, and the rash feels rough and gravel-like to the touch. It is more common in teenage boys than girls and is very rarely seen in adults. The pimples are more on the face, and very close to the hairline on the forehead and temples. If this is true, it might be aggravated by the use of hair gel and spray, together with sweat. The skin is generally pale and somewhat thin.

TRADITIONAL CHINESE MEDICINE VIEW

- Pale, thin skin – Lung Blood and yin deficiency.
- Many little red papules with none or very few yellow heads.
- Papules may bleed when picked by the patient.
- Healed papules leave no scars, and skin returns to smooth again.
- Papules may itch.

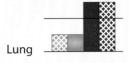

Lung

TREATMENT

- Tonify Lung yin – Lu 1, Lu 7, Ren 17 (needled in direction to face).

- Sedate Lung yang – LI 2 sedation.

- Purify Blood and cool heat – Sp 10, UB 17.

- Wind elimination sedation on GB 20 and other suitable points.

- Drink more water, eat white rice, sleep more, avoid coffee.

- Usually three or four sessions make a substantial difference, at two sessions per week. Treatment can be terminated after this, or repeated once or twice a month if necessary (Figure 6.4).

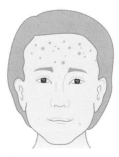

Figure 6.4 Acne like 'prickly heat'

As with the treatment of acne rosacea, there are no local points used except if there are pustules. The main treatment is to tonify the yin and, if there are symptoms of Blood deficiency, to tonify the Blood. The treatment stated is so effective that one sees changes in the red colour of the papules before the needles are removed after the first treatment.

6.3 PSORIASIS

Psoriasis is a normal papulosquamous disorder affecting 2 per cent of the population and is characterized by well-demarcated red, scaly plaques. The skin becomes inflamed and hyperproliferates at about ten times the normal rate. It affects males and females equally. The ages of onset are 16–22 years (early onset) and 55–60 years (late onset). Early-onset psoriasis is more common.

I describe two types of psoriasis below (Figure 6.5).

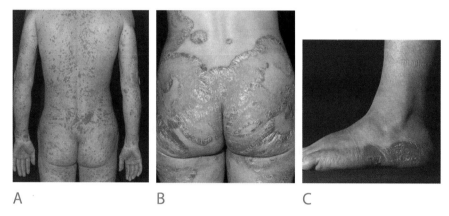

A   B   C

Figure 6.5 (A–C) Psoriasis

6.3.1 Damp-cold type psoriasis

WESTERN MEDICAL CONCEPT

Guttate psoriasis

'Raindrop-like' psoriasis is a variant most commonly seen in children and young adults. It may start explosively after a streptococcal sore throat, when very small circular or oval plaques appear over the trunk.

Chronic plaque psoriasis

This is the most common type of psoriasis. It is characterized by pinkish-red scaly plaques, especially on extensor surfaces such as knees and elbows. The lower back, ears and scalp are also commonly involved. New plaques of psoriasis occur at sites of skin trauma.

DAMP-COLD TYPE PSORIASIS – TRADITIONAL CHINESE MEDICINE VIEW

- Raised, rough and reddened areas covered with fine, silvery scales.
- The scales are shed all the time, covering bedding and clothes.
- For a short time after a bath the skin becomes more red and less scaly.
- The condition worsens in winter and improves in summer, especially in warm sea water.
- The patient is affected by the appearance of the skin rather than itching or discomfort.
- During healing, the skin first becomes depigmented, and then changes to normal colour.

TREATMENT

- Small area – meridian 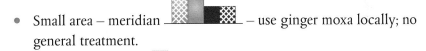 – use ginger moxa locally; no general treatment.

- Large area – Lung  – UB 13, LI 11, Lu 10.

- Extensive – use LI 4, St 25, TW 6, St 40 and Sp 9; also use Lu 5 sedation; no smoking.

- The more extensive the psoriasis, the more difficult it is to treat. Ginger moxa locally on the lesions, regular baths in highly salted water and sunlight are all helpful. Treatment is best given in a course of 12–14 sessions; the initial course can involve bi-weekly treatments, and later courses can be once a week.

Damp-cold-type psoriasis is dormant in nature – it does not cause any irritation or itching, but looks bad. Common areas affected include the backs of elbows and fronts of knees, and it can often be associated with arthritis. This type of psoriasis responds well to acupuncture, especially if the patches are small and few. The treatment principle is to circulate and eliminate the dampness, and warm the affected areas. If there are only one or two patches they can be treated with ginger moxa alone, without needles. The technique is described in detail on page 113. The larger the area, the more important it becomes to eliminate dampness – points Sp 9 and Lu 5 descend dampness to eliminate it; and smaller areas only need to warm and circulate the dampness.

Points UB 13, LI 11 and Lu 10 are for tonifying the yang and Qi of the Lung. UB 13 is the Back-Shu point of the Lung; LI 11 is the tonification point of the coupled organ; and Lu 10 is the fire point/grandmother point of the Lung, and this tonifies the yang aspect of the Lung.

Local needling is also very effective in this type of psoriasis. On the normal skin, subcutaneous punctures can be used around the affected patches. The idea is to increase blood circulation around the area (the same principle as moxa). It is therefore necessary that the patient cooperates to reduce the dampness by following a strict diet.

6.3.2 Damp-heat type psoriasis

WESTERN MEDICAL CONCEPT

Flexural psoriasis

This tends to occur in later life. It is characterized by well-demarcated, red, glazed plaques confined to flexures such as the groin, natal cleft and submammary area. There is less scaling.

Erythrodermic and pustular psoriasis

These are the most severe types of psoriasis, reflecting a widespread inflammation of the skin. They may be associated with fever, malaise and circulatory disturbances.

They are more localized variants of pustular psoriasis that confine themselves to hands and feet but they are not associated with severe systemic symptoms. These types are more common in heavy cigarette smokers.

In my experience, this type of psoriasis is more difficult to treat effectively than the previous type. It is more extensive, and both the skin generally and that of the psoriasis is thicker and does not respond well to needle stimulation. If these patients are smokers – as they often are – treatment will not be effective at all. I always ask these patients if they are smokers before we start acupuncture, and tell them that unless they stop, the acupuncture will not work for them. They have to make a decision before treatment begins.

> ## DAMP-HEAT TYPE PSORIASIS – TRADITIONAL CHINESE MEDICINE VIEW
>
> - Thick, hard and raised reddish areas with white scales.
> - Pruritus with bleeding or inflammation.
> - Patches appear on arms, legs, torso, neck and scalp.
> - Patches tend to wander and spread fast.
>
> Damp-heat in Lung

TREATMENT

- This type is treated similar to damp-heat type neurodermatitis.

- General points – Sp 10, UB 17, Du 20, SI 8 sedation, TW 10 sedation.

- For elimination and circulation of dampness – LI 4, St 25, TW 6 and Sp 9, St 40, Lu 5.

- To eliminate heat: either dispersing heat technique (see page 102) or local plum-blossom tapping to bleed; Lu 5 venous bleeding.

- Avoid milk products, fatty foods and refined sugars.

- Avoid coffee and alcohol; reduce consumption of red meat.

- Treatment twice weekly for eight sessions, then once weekly for six to eight sessions, then reduce frequency gradually.

The treatment is to eliminate dampness, but also to disperse heat. The points SI 8 and TW 10 are used to sedate the yang of the Heart and pericardium indirectly, through their coupled organs. Lu 5 bleeding, plum-blossom tapping to bleed local patches or dispersing fire needle technique (see page 102) can be used to disperse heat.

The points LI 4, St 25 and TW 6, which are the constipation points, and Sp 9 and Lu 5, which are points to descend dampness to the urinary system, will get rid of excessive dampness from the body. Point St 40 should circulate any stagnating fluid.

The next possible method to push the improvement forward would be to bleed distally, either on the finger- or toe-tip or the jing-well point of the meridian where the psoriasis is present, or on a vein that is distal to the lesion but still along the same longitudinal line.

ADVICE FOR PATIENTS

Between dampness and heat, the dampness seems to be the underlying cause, and the heat seems to be caused by the stagnant dampness. It is therefore necessary that the patient cooperates with us to reduce the dampness by following a strict diet. As the dampness always comes from the Spleen to the skin, there is no easy way to achieve this other than by reducing all damp-producing foods and heavy evening meals. When the dampness diminishes, the heat will reduce of its own accord.

Light cotton clothing and exposure to wind or fresh air when possible will assist the movement of damp stagnation. Baths in sea water, or home-prepared high-saline baths will remove dampness through osmosis, and are very good to take once or twice weekly.

With all of these additional therapies, one could achieve fairly good results with the acupuncture. There may be an improvement of 50–75 per cent after 12 to 14 treatment sessions. The yang areas such as the scalp, neck, arms and torso are the first to clear; the yin regions such as the buttocks, inguinal area and the legs clear more slowly. After achieving about 50 per cent improvement, some local treatment on the stubborn patches may be advisable (Figure 6.6).

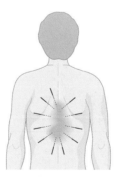

Figure 6.6 Local needling around area of psoriasis

6.4 WARTS

WESTERN MEDICAL CONCEPT

Warts are small solid growths, arising from the surface of the skin. They are usually due to a papillomavirus infection of the skin. They typically disappear after a few months but can last for years and can recur. They are highly infectious, and it is estimated that 10 per cent of the population suffer from them. The infection is most likely to be spread in schools by hand-holding games, and among adolescents by walking barefoot on gymnasium floors and around swimming pools (Figure 6.7).

Warts come in various sizes and shapes, alone or in hundreds.

Common warts develop on the skin of children and young people on the knuckles, on the backs of the hands and on the knees. Occasionally such warts come out in a crop. In structure, they consist of a bundle of fibres produced by overgrowth of the papillae in the true skin, each bundle enveloped by a cap of the horny cells that cover the surface of the epidermis, and the whole mass being surrounded by a ring of thickened epidermis.

Flat warts, which are flat-topped, are most common on the face and the backs of the hands.

Plantar warts occur on the soles of the feet, most commonly in older children and adolescents.

Soft warts, consisting of little tags of skin, are found especially upon the neck, chest, ears or eyelids of people whose skin has been subjected for a long time to some irritation.

Genital warts occur in the genital area.

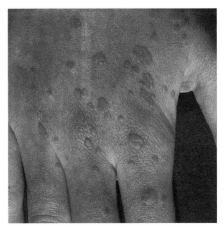

A

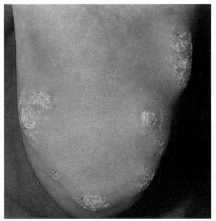

B

Figure 6.7 Warts

CASE STUDY

A 14-year-old boy was brought to see me by his father, one of the doctors who had attended my acupuncture course, where we talked about the effectiveness of acupuncture as a treatment for warts. The patient had extremely large warts covering his entire palms and soles. They resembled large vesicles rather than solid forms, extending over the sides of the palms and soles. He was very self-conscious about these, and sat on his hands and hid his feet.

We decided that he had excessive dampness on the skin, and also in the Spleen – as both the hands and feet were affected, and the Spleen is responsible for the peripheral circulation of body fluid. We used Sp 9, St 40 and UB 20 to improve the dampness in the Spleen, and applied ginger moxa to the hands and feet. On his hands he had thin slices of ginger smoking with moxa wool, and on the feet we rubbed the skin with fresh ginger and then warmed the area with a moxa cigar.

The father was tasked with continuing this treatment but, like all doctors, was too busy to carry out the treatment as frequently as he should. The boy received only one treatment every 2 weeks when he should have had at least two treatments a week. Despite this, his skin cleared completely within a few weeks, and when I saw him after 6 months he was totally cured.

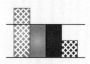

WARTS – TRADITIONAL CHINESE MEDICINE VIEW

- A stagnation of damp on meridian if it is in a small area (e.g. dorsum of hand).
- Damp stagnation in Lung if they are extensive.

Treatment

- Local needles around wart or hot needle in the wart.
- Local moxa or ginger moxa – tonify yang, sedate yin of meridian.
- Two treatments weekly, 8–12 sessions in total.

Treatment of plantar warts – foot sole is associated with the Kidneys

- UB 58 Luo-connecting point.
- UB 23 Back-Shu point.
- Ginger moxa on sole, over the warts.
- If extensive, sedate Lu 5.

Warts are common among children and adolescents. They occur mostly on the hands and face. They are infectious and can spread easily. All soft and common warts are easy to treat, and it is sufficient to treat small warts only locally. The best local treatment is moxa, and the effect of the moxa may be enhanced by ginger – either thin slices on which the moxa wool is placed and lit to smoke, or fresh ginger rubbed on the wart and then a moxa cigar held to the skin. One or two needles placed subcutaneously very close to the wart before moxa is given would also be good. The idea is to increase Blood and Qi flow in the area, so that the stagnation is eliminated. Local treatment should be carried out daily by the patient or a family member. Usually, the warts will disappear on their own after 8–12 treatments, but this may occur only after treatment is completed.

Special local treatment – fire needle

I learned and witnessed this technique many times during my studies in China. It was done on many cold tumours, thyroid tumours and warts. It seemed to shrink the tumour (but not cause it to disappear altogether) within days. But the technique left the patient with blood streaming down the skin (not when treating warts), which was a very unpleasant experience. When you read about the technique, you will understand why I no longer use it on my patients.

THE TECHNIQUE

Take a metal-handled needle and, wrapping the handle in gauze to protect your hand, hold the tip of the needle (about 1–1.5 cm) in a fire (we used a spirit burner). When the needle is red hot, quickly puncture the wart with the tip and then withdraw the needle immediately. You will hear the skin sizzle. This is done only once for each wart. The wart will gradually dry and shrink to disappear over the next few days.

6.4.1 Plantar warts

The example given in the previous box is for treating plantar warts. As the foot sole is mainly associated with the Kidneys, the problem is treated as a damp stagnation of the Kidney. The Qi is tonified by K 3, the grandmother point, which tonifies the Kidney yang aspect, and UB 23, the Back-Shu point. UB 58, the Luo-connecting point, is used in order to make the shift – to sedate yin and tonify yang simultaneously.

6.4.2 Warts on the dorsum of the hand

If the warts are mainly on the back of the hands, then we could treat the Triple Warmer meridian. The points we would use are UB 22 (Back-Shu of the Triple Warmer), TW 6 (house element point) and TW 5 (Luo-connecting point).

6.4.3 Warts on the palms

If the warts are mainly on the palm, then we should be treating the Lung meridian, as this flows on the palm. We can use points UB 13 (Back-Shu of Lung), Lu 10 (the grandmother point) and LI 6 (Luo-connecting point).[1]

> If the warts are extensive and cover many meridians, then sedation of Lung yin with point Lu 5, the sedation point, is necessary.

6.5 ALOPECIA

> ### WESTERN MEDICAL CONCEPT
> Researchers have determined that this form of hair loss is related to hormones called androgens, particularly an androgen called dihydrotestosterone.
>
> Androgens are important for normal male sexual development before birth and during puberty. Androgens also have other important functions in both males and females, such as regulating hair growth and sex drive.

There are various types of alopecia. A common pattern of male hair loss is that it begins above both temples or at the vertex, and may progress to complete baldness (Figure 6.8). In women, the hair usually becomes thin all over the head, and the hairline does not recede.

Our head hair is nourished by Kidney yin and Liver Blood. Thinning or loss of hair occurs when one is overworked or stressed, when there is blood loss or anaemia, or when the climate is very dry. Dryness makes the hair brittle and causes split ends. Blood deficiency (also due to stress and overwork, because stress consumes Liver Blood) makes the roots weak,

---

1 Note that if you want to shift the energy from yin to yang (sedate yin and tonify yang) with an element, it is always the Luo connecting point of the yang meridian that is used.

and the individual strands of hair thin and dull. The mechanical strain of washing, combing or even moving the head on the pillow is enough to cause the loss of large handfuls of hair. When treating hair loss, it is necessary to nourish and moisten the hair, and it will flourish again in growth. It is important to initiate treatment as soon as symptoms develop as, once complete baldness sets in, it will be very difficult to make a difference.

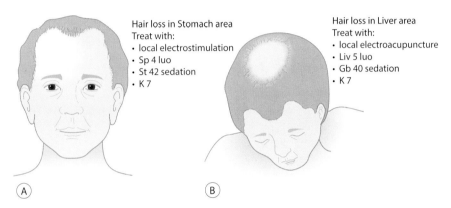

Hair loss in Stomach area
Treat with:
• local electrostimulation
• Sp 4 luo
• St 42 sedation
• K 7

Hair loss in Liver area
Treat with:
• local electroacupuncture
• Liv 5 luo
• Gb 40 sedation
• K 7

(A)　　　　(B)

Figure 6.8 Alopecia in different head regions.
(A) Hair loss in Stomach area; (B) hair loss in Liver area

I have addressed general hair loss and partial hair loss on certain areas of the head as the two types of hair loss that give good results with acupuncture. Both energy treatment and local treatment is given. The patient should take some vitamin–amino acid combinations such as Panthovigar N®, which contains thiamine, calcium pantothenate, cystine and keratin, and carry out some local care.

TRADITIONAL CHINESE MEDICINE VIEW

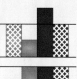 Hyperactive yang in meridian (excessive heat in head area)

 Liver Blood deficiency

 Kidney yin deficiency

Four head areas

Front and temples	Stomach, Large Intestine
Vertex	Liver, Pericardium
Side	Gall Bladder, Triple Warmer
Occiput	Urinary Bladder, Small Intestine

Local treatment

Electrostimulation or plum-blossom tapping to bleed
Point K 7, drink water and rest
Sedate yang and tonify yin of specific head area.

EXPLAINING THE TREATMENT

In hair loss of any type, *the Kidney yin must first be tonified, ideally on point K 7*. The patient should also drink water more regularly and rest more. Where possible, a midday rest would be excellent, as midday is the worst time energetically for those who have Kidney yin deficiency. If Kidney yin is deficient, this would generate uncontrolled Kidney yang, which rises to the head.

If *Liver Blood deficiency* can be established, then the Blood should be tonified with points Ren 14, UB 15, UB 17, Sp 10, GB 39 and an iron supplement.

The next thing to do would be the local treatment. This is done (1) in the area with hair loss, and (2) on the organs associated with the areas of the hair loss.

6.5.1 Local treatment on the area of hair loss

This area should be examined well. If there is some hair and the scalp has normal roughness, then electrical stimulation should be used. This will cool the scalp in the area.

THE TECHNIQUE – ELECTRICAL STIMULATION ON AREA OF HAIR LOSS

The area with thinning hair is treated with four subcutaneous needles, two on each side, and these are connected to two outlets of an electrical stimulator (taking care to connect the two needles on the same side of the body to one outlet). The needles are then stimulated at a continuous frequency, around 10 Hz, for 20 minutes.

This needling is relatively painful, and is therefore difficult to repeat more than twice weekly for 2 weeks, and then has to be done once weekly for a further four to eight sessions (Figure 6.9).

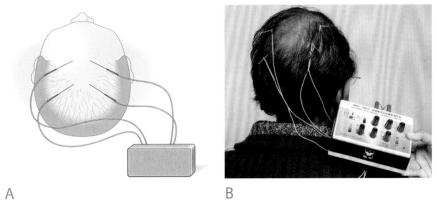

A   B

Figure 6.9 Electrical stimulation to cool the area of hair loss

When there is no hair at all in the affected area, this area can be treated locally with plum-blossom tapping to bleed. The tapping therapy has to be done daily for up to 14 days. It would be more convenient and practical for the patient to take a plum-blossom hammer home and get a family member to do it for them (Figure 6.10).

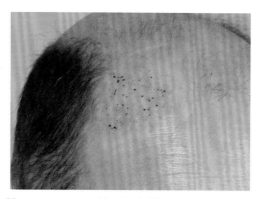

Figure 6.10 Plum-blossom tapping to bleed in bald areas

THE TECHNIQUE – PLUM-BLOSSOM TAPPING ON BALD AREA

Clean the area well with surgical spirit and allow it to dry. Holding the plum-blossom hammer, tap hard vertically on the bald area in no particular direction. When finished, this area should be covered with droplets of blood, which should be wiped off.

This treatment is very effective for small areas of baldness, or in alopecia areata. It is not as successful for large areas or if the entire head is bald. Within 14 days of treatment, one can see and feel fluff-like hair growing in this area. The initial growth is grey coloured, and is not the colour of the rest of the hair. But within 1–3 months the hair will become thicker and more coloured. Once the 'fluff' starts to appear, the bleeding tapping should be stopped. Local treatment is no longer necessary. If needed, electrostimulation could be given (Figure 6.9).

6.5.2 Treatment on the organs associated with hair loss

The common areas for hair loss are the temples and vertex. In alopecia areata, it can be anywhere on the head. There is empirical knowledge that different parts of the head are related to different organs of the body, and that imbalances of these particular organs will manifest as pain, hair loss, greying or skin problems in these parts of the head.

According to the box on page 150, the frontal head (including both temples) is associated with the Stomach and Large Intestine, the bright yang organs. Headache that is due to hunger or low blood sugar will occur in this area. A headache that accompanies gastritis will also manifest in this area. Hair loss in this area is due to excessive heat in the Stomach or Large Intestine (more often the Stomach). Just as hair grows more in areas that are cold, to insulate and protect these areas, so the body will lose hair in areas that are hot, in an attempt to keep cool.

Thus, hair loss occurring only in the area of the Stomach or Large Intestine needs to be treated by balancing the energy there – tonifying the yin and sedating the yang (the yin needs to be tonified, because this is a long-term imbalance and there will be some deficiencies too – as there is heat, the deficiency must be with the yin aspect).

ENERGY-BALANCING POINTS FOR FRONTAL HAIR LOSS

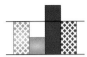 Balance Stomach yin deficiency and yang excess

- Ren 12 – Front-mu of Stomach (will cool and calm the Stomach).

- Sp 4 and St 42 sedation – combining the Luo-connecting point of the yin organ and sedation of the yuan-source point of the yang organ will tonify yin and sedate yang.

- Take care with diet – avoid foods that may irritate the Stomach and increase heat – mainly alcohol, strong coffee and spices.

ENERGY-BALANCING POINTS FOR VERTEX HAIR LOSS

 Balance Liver yin deficiency and yang excess

- Liv 5 and GB 40 sedation – Luo-connecting point of yin organ and sedate the yuan-source point of yang organ.

- Avoid sour foods, alcohol and stress, all of which will increase the Liver yang aspect.

In the case of both hair loss and premature greying of head hair (the second is a symptom of Kidney yang deficiency), patients seem to express concern only when it is too late. In traditional Chinese medicine, we worry about tendencies of the body rather than extreme symptoms, predominantly because the more chronic and far gone an imbalance, the more difficult it becomes to correct. When imbalances are detected early, however, they are easier to correct and prevent from going into a chronic state.

It is normal to lose hair during climate changes and when the weather is dry, during at least two cycles of the year. But then the hair grows again and returns to the earlier state. If one notices hair loss in large quantities –

covering the pillow or the shower base – it is alarmingly high and needs treatment. Because, even if hair grows again, it will be thinner than before and there will be less of it. If we notice hair loss when we are overworked, when we have long periods of poor sleep and when we are generally run down, then we need to treat the hair loss.

6.5.3 Hair loss – dos and don'ts

- Gently massage the scalp with coconut, olive or sesame oil, leave it on for 30 minutes or overnight, and then wash. This will cool and nourish the hair roots and is much better than any conditioner; this can be done once a week.

- Take a multivitamin product.

- Take a herbal iron supplement if there is Blood deficiency.

- Go to bed before midnight.

- Post-menopausal women, or men of the same age, should have an afternoon rest whenever possible (the heat tends to rise up because of the Kidney yin deficiency).

- Drink plenty of water regularly. Eat watery foods and greens.

- Keep the head cool (not cold!). If one has a hot head and cold feet, then a warm foot bath will change this order.

- Don't wash hair too often – twice weekly is fine. If hair is too greasy, there is a fault with the diet. This can be caused by excessive milk products, cheese, processed meats such as sausage, fatty meats and oily preparations and excessive refined sugars.

- Avoid close caps and hats when possible: they increase the damp-heat in the head.

- The hairdryer is not a plumping machine for a head with less hair! It dries and scorches the roots. Do not use a hairdryer regularly unless it is necessary to go out soon after washing the hair – and then keep it at a reasonable distance. Ask your hairdresser (who uses it too close to the scalp) to do the same.

- Avoid direct sunlight on the head for long. Carry an umbrella if you need to stand in the sun.

- Avoid coffee and alcohol.

6.6   HYPERHIDROSIS

Hyperhidrosis is a condition characterized by abnormally increased perspiration, in excess of that required for regulation of body temperature, and is a major problem for many patients, who often undergo some kind of treatment. Sufferers feel a loss of control because perspiration takes place independent of temperature and emotional state. Acupuncture is effective in these cases, especially when patients sweat all over the body.

Hyperhidrosis can be primary or secondary. Secondary hyperhidrosis can start at any point in life, and may be due to a disorder of the thyroid or pituitary gland, diabetes mellitus, tumours, gout, menopause or certain drugs. Anxiety, certain foods and drinks, nicotine, caffeine and smells can trigger a response.

Hyperhidrosis can be generalized or localized to specific parts of the body. The hands, feet, axillae and the groin area are the most active regions because of the relatively high concentration of sweat glands in these areas.

Hyperhidrosis is treated quite aggressively in Western medicine, often with botulinum (botox) injections. Following these injections, patients will experience compensatory hyperhidrosis in areas other than those that have been suppressed.

Hyperhidrosis is a condition that responds reasonably well to acupuncture, and it works better for larger areas than smaller (such as axillae). The key issue is to decide if it is a hot or cold problem to begin with.

6.6.1 Hot sweating

If there is heat, it is normal to sweat, and the therapy should be to disperse heat with sedation or cool the heat with yin tonification. These patients have a red complexion, feel hot and restless and suffer from excessive sweating. The tongue and pulse show signs of heat and, if there is yin deficiency, concentrated urine and hard stools will also be symptoms.

- If the heat and sweating are due to yin deficiency, then they will be intermittent, and worse at night-time and during sleep (because the yin improves at this time, and they have sufficient fluid to sweat with).

- If the heat and sweating are more or less permanent and worse during activity or talking, that is when the yang is high.

Explaining the points

POINTS FOR HOT SWEATING

- General points – Lu 7, K 7 (Lu 7 is used to close the skin pores and K 7 is used for holding the water in the body).

- For sweating of hands and upper body (Heart and Lung):

  o SI 8 sedation (to sedate Heart yang indirectly).

  o He 5 and SI 2 (to tonify Heart yin and Small Intestine yin).

  o Ren 14 and Sp 6 (to tonify Heart and general yin).

  o LI 2 sedation (indirect sedation of Lung yang).

TABLE 6.3 EXCESSIVE HOT SWEATING – THERAPY PLAN[*]

General points: Lu 7, K 7		
Hands and upper body		
Hyperactive yang or yang excess in Heart and Lung		SI 8 sedation, **H 5**, **SI 2**, **Ren 14**, Sp 6 (for Heart), LI 2 sedation, bleed Lu 5, **Lu 1**, **Ren 17** (for Lung)
Feet and lower body (smelly feet)		
Hyperactive yang in Kidney		**K 7** or **K 10**, Sp 6, **UB 40**, **Ren 3**
Hands and feet (red, warm and wet)		
Damp-heat in Spleen		UB 20/UB 21 dispersing heat technique
		Ren 12, P 6, Liv 3
		Avoid heat-producing foods such as red meat or fish, coffee, alcohol and spicy or bitter flavours

[*] *The points in bold have a yin tonification effect.*

- ○ Bleed or use dispersing heat technique on Lu 5 (to eliminate Lung heat).

- ○ Lu 1, Lu 7 (to tonify Lung yin).

- For hot sweating of feet and lower body (including genitals – hot sweating in these areas is due to yin deficiency heat and therefore tends to be smelly):

  - ○ K 7 (tonifies Kidney yin).

  - ○ K 10 (tonifies Kidney yin).

  - ○ Only one of the two points above should be used in one session.

  - ○ Sp 6 (tonifies the three yin meridians of the leg).

  - ○ Ren 3 (Front-mu point of Urinary Bladder – tonifies yin).

  - ○ B1 40 (tonifies Urinary Bladder yin over the grandmother – Spleen).

- For hot sweating of hands and feet (this is generally together with dampness, and therefore the sweat is sticky and the extremities warm and slightly swollen):

  - ○ B1 20 or B1 21 heat elimination technique (to eliminate heat).

  - ○ Ren 12 (Front-mu of Stomach – cools and calms).

  - ○ P 6 (distal point of upper abdomen – also calming).

  - ○ Liv 3 (calms Stomach yang).

ADVICE FOR PATIENTS

When treating hot sweating, it might be useful to discuss the patient's lifestyle and eating habits. Patients do not always associate their output with their input.

- It may be helpful if they avoid hot baths and reduce the temperature of the shower. Avoid saunas or Turkish baths.

- Heat-producing foods such as red meat, shellfish, coffee and especially alcohol and spicy and bitter-flavoured foods should be avoided.

- Patients should cultivate a habit of sipping water throughout the day, not drinking a whole bottle when they remember.

- Synthetic fibres should be avoided as much as possible and cotton fabric used for clothes.

- With the consent of their partner, they could keep their bedroom cool – this would help the yin to be tonified through the night. If night sweating can be avoided, then the yin has a chance to recover.

6.6.2 Cold sweating

While hot sweating tends to be on larger areas of the body, cold sweating occurs on smaller areas such as the extremities. The patients are often cold in the whole or in part of the body, pale, and have a pale or blue tongue. It is interesting that the sweating is usually in the coldest part of the body, at the extremities. The sweat is watery and without smell or stickiness. It can happen all day long, though it is noticeably less when the patient is asleep. Here, we have two problems to treat:

- the coldness.

- the sweating – it is not normal to sweat when one is cold. The fact that this is so suggests a Lung Qi deficiency, where the Lung has lost control over the function of the skin pores.

TABLE **6.4** EXCESSIVE COLD SWEATING – THERAPY PLAN

General points: UB 13, LI 11, Lu 7		
Hands		
Heart Blood, yang and Qi deficiency		Ren 14, UB 15, H 9, SI 3, Lu 9 (Influential point for blood vessels)
Lung Qi deficiency		UB 13, LI 11
Feet		
Kidney yin and yang deficiency		K 7, UB 67, K 1 moxa, Lu 9

Hands and feet		
Spleen Blood, yang and Qi deficiency		Liv 13, UB 20, St 36, Lu 9, moxa on Sp 1, Ren 12, P 8, K 1
		Eat cooked and warm food, and drink warm fluids

Patients with cold sweating do not like to overdress, because they feel everything gets wet with sweat. It might be an idea to dress warmly on the arms and legs – right up to the wrists and ankles. Those with sweaty hands and feet will also have to eat and drink warm substances, so as to keep their middle warm.

In my experience, hot sweating responds better to acupuncture than cold sweating, probably because in the first case the problem is not the sweating but the heat. In the case of cold sweating, the main problem seems to be the Lung Qi deficiency, because the skin is open when it should be closed. But if it is only a Lung Qi deficiency, the sweating should occur all over. Here, the sweating occurs only in the cold areas of the body. Therefore, it is also necessary to treat the cold.

CASE STUDY

A 28-year-old man was treated on one of my courses in Germany for the complaint of smelly feet. This is a not uncommon complaint in young men who participate in sport, but in this particular patient it was a major problem. His feet would smell even immediately after a bath in scented water and he did not wear shoes. He had no girlfriend.

The patient was a warm person with slight hair loss. We decided to tonify his Kidney yin. He was asked to drink more water. We first decided on a few points, but soon realized that he had a needle phobia. So we settled on one single point on each leg – this was K 10 (own-element point). We treated him daily – his friend who participated in the course gave the needles. The patient fainted or came very near to fainting each time we treated him. But he wanted to continue the treatment. After the tenth session, the smell was gone.

For this patient, all the fainting was worthwhile!

CASE STUDY

A 67-year-old man was another case brought to one of my courses in Germany. His niece was his guest during the time she was participating in the course, and when she heard of his problem she wanted to help him.

This patient experienced severe sweating, principally on his upper body, head, chest and arms, all the time. This was very much worse when he was talking. He was quite red in his face and had diabetes. His problem had started in his later life, though he was not quite sure exactly when. He had the problem for more than 3 years before treatment.

We decided that the problem was chronic and we should therefore treat some deficiency as well. Since this was hot sweating and a yang-dominant state, the yin must have been deficient.

We tonified his general yin and gave him Heart and Lung yang sedation.

We used the following points: Ren 17, Ren 14, Ren 3 and Lu 7 (this combination is also for tonifying the Ren meridian to tonify the general yin of body); sedate SI 8 and sedate TW 10 (to sedate the yang of fire element); Lu 7 (to close the skin and tonify Lung yin); and K 7 to tonify the Kidney yin in order to control the yang of the fire element.

In just three treatment sessions he had improved considerably. I did not have the opportunity of meeting him after that, so I am unable to tell you the end result of the treatment.

6.7 URTICARIA

Both acute and chronic urticaria are of an allergic origin. Common causes of allergy are contact with metals or dyes and consumption of shellfish, nuts, eggs, fish, acid or derivatives. It is also common as a drug allergy (Figure 6.11).

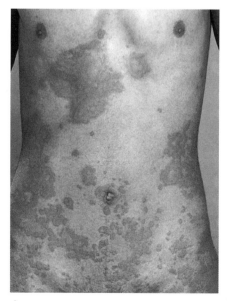

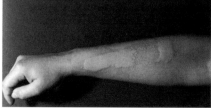

A

B

Figure 6.11 Urticaria

The skin lesions of urticarial disease are caused by an inflammatory reaction in the skin causing leakage from the capillaries in the epidermis, resulting in an oedema that persists until the fluid has been absorbed into the surrounding cells. The skin manifests raised and red weals, which itch severely.

Urticaria is a typical wind-heat symptom of the Lung. It is easier to cure if it is acute and recurrent, and somewhat more difficult when it is a chronic state. It is easier to make a difference in a situation that is changing or changeable, rather than one that is constant. With acute urticaria, one is able to improve the situation within 10 to 20 minutes.

In a recurrent urticaria that occurs due to food or contact, it is possible to increase tolerance. In chronic urticaria, one needs at least six to eight sessions before any change can be expected.

CASE STUDY

This female patient (aged 34) was the wife of a diplomat in one of the embassies in Sri Lanka. She was allergic to many metals – including her wedding ring, which she could not wear. She could not take her car keys in her hand, or use metal cutlery. If she did, she would develop severe urticaria in and around that area. Being a diplomat's wife, she had to attend many dinners, and she felt very embarrassed to have to take her wooden-handled cutlery with her!

After 12 treatments, she was able to wear her wedding ring up to 3 days in a row. She was able to eat with metal forks and hold her car keys. So although the tendency was still present, the tolerance had increased.

A treatment plan for acute urticaria is described below.

- Wind-heat in Lung – pruritus, inflammation.

- Skin thickness and moisture depends on quantity of dampness and yin.

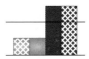

- Acute urticaria – wind-heat in Lung.

- Points: Lu 6 sedation[2], LI 2 sedation, Sp 10, Lu 5 venous bleeding.

- If symptoms are not gone, then add SI 8 and TW 10 sedation and Du 20.

> Treatment should be given twice weekly in both recurrent and chronic urticaria for 5 weeks. The course may be repeated in 3 months or so, which generally has a very good effect.

TABLE 6.5 URTICARIA

Recurrent urticaria	Chronic urticaria
No symptoms in interval	Some level of symptoms
Dry-heat in Lung	Damp-heat in Lung
Points given during interval: Lu 1 or Lu 8, Ren 17, P 6; LI 2 sedation; Sp 10 or UB 17; Sp 6 descending technique if problem only in upper body	Points given at any time: Lu 5, Sp 9, St 40; Sp 10 or UB 17; LI 4, St 25, TW 6 (for elimination)
Dermagraphia test on ventral forearm produces a prolonged white line	Dermagraphia causes instant red weal

6.8 VITILIGO

Vitiligo or leukoderma is a chronic skin condition that causes a loss of pigment, resulting in irregular pale patches of skin. Most cases occur before the age of 20, and the condition can worsen and cover a large extent of the skin very quickly or remain constant in size. It often appears symmetrically across both sides of the body. This is a disease where the yang and Qi do not ascend to the skin because they are both deficient (Figure 6.12).

---

2 In acute urticaria, the Lu 6 sedation needle must be vibrated often. The needles generally stay in for 20–30 minutes; the vibration should be done every 5 minutes.

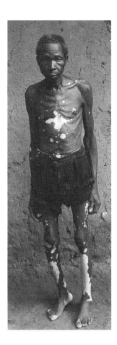

Figure 6.12 Vitiligo

Back in Sri Lanka, my clinic was full of vitiligo patients – it was much worse for patients with dark skin to show white patches than for those with lighter skin! Acupuncture treatment was so successful that I had dermatologists from all over the country coming to learn the treatment. We found that older vitiligo patches (over 1½ years–2 years) did not respond to treatment, but the newer areas responded within 2 weeks. We also had the patients take part in the treatment – when they developed any new patches they could attack them instantly.

The treatment principle is to bring the yang and Qi back to the surface of the skin.

The following is the body treatment plan for vitiligo.

VITILIGO – DEPIGMENTATION

Local treatment – ginger moxa or plum-blossom tapping until red, daily for 14 days.

 Energy balance – of the meridian where it manifests

This should be tonified if, for example:

- The eyelids are affected, then Spleen yang should be tonified with UB 20, Sp 1 and St 41
- Dorsum of hands are affected, TW 3, UB 22 should be tonified

 If vitiligo is extensive, then Lung is affected

- Points used – UB 13, LI 11, Lu 10, SI 3

 If worsening rapidly, then Lung is affected

- Points used – Lu 1, Lu 9, UB 13, LI 11, perhaps also Sp 3 and St 36

In the last case, the treatment might help only to stop the spreading, and repigment the most recent patches.

When treating vitiligo, the local treatment was found to be the most effective. This was mainly ginger moxa or plum-blossom tapping. But in vitiligo of the eyelids, both these therapies were unsuitable. Where patients had other affected areas and also depigmentation of eyelids, we performed local treatment on the other areas and the general points and did not treat the eyelids. Even in these cases, the skin around the eyelids became pigmented again.

6.8.1 The technique for local treatment

Ginger moxa

Cut fresh ginger into slices approximately 1/8 cm thick, punch many needle-holes in the slices, and place these slices on the vitiligo patches. Take loose moxa wool and spread it thinly on the ginger slices. Light the moxa in many places and let it burn slowly. If the heat is uncomfortable, the ginger slices can be moved between areas, or removed altogether. When the slices are removed, the vitiligo patch should be red in colour.

Plum-blossom tapping

Tap with the plum-blossom hammer on the vitiligo patch until it is red. The tapping should be controlled so as not to produce bleeding.

Both local treatments can be used on a patient. Generally speaking, one patch is treated throughout with one method. The patches on the face are treated with tapping because moxa is contraindicated near mucous membranes. The local treatment is given daily for up to 14 days. Small dots of hyperpigmentation will form within the vitiligo patches in this time. The patient should be told about this, lest they get worried about a third colour appearing! These darker dots will diffuse and cover the vitiligo patch.

The patient can carry on the local treatment at home over the next 14 days and then whenever they notice a new patch appearing. A complete new patch will disappear within 3–4 days of daily treatment.

CASE STUDY

One of the numerous vitiligo patients in my clinic in Sri Lanka was a young boy. I am not sure if he was 6 or 8 years old because he was quite small in size but communicated to us with the wisdom of an adult. He had started having small patches of vitiligo 6 months previously. Within just 6 months his entire lower legs were milky white. He then began to develop small patches on the rest of the body.

This was a serious case, requiring serious measures. We decided that, in addition to the Lung being severely deficient, the rest of the body had very little yang and Qi. I am sure that his Spleen Blood (general nutritional state) was deficient too, but this was not an issue we could address with needles. Because he was a child, we did not want to give many needles. Local treatment was impossible, considering the extent of the problem. We gave him Lu 9 and LI 11 and Du channel tonification. The Du channel is the most yang meridian of the body, and tonifying the Du will amount to tonifying the entire yang energy of the body. To make this even more effective and painless, we decided to do moxa on the Du meridian.

Instead of placing ginger slices on this little boy, we rubbed the Du meridian with wet ginger slices, and then moved a moxa cigar from coccyx to hairline, in the direction of energy flow, until the skin had a red reaction. We treated him daily except at weekends. Within ten sessions, more than 50 per cent of the skin on his lower legs had recovered its pigmentation. This was truly a fantastic result for such a simple treatment. The boy was a patient in my clinic for a long time, as I asked him to return from time to time for a set of booster treatments. He was completely cured within 6 months, and if he noticed any new patches he could treat them locally by himself. He also acted as my pacifier for new younger patients who did not like needles.

6.9 HYPERPIGMENTATION

Hyperpigmentation is the opposite of vitiligo, where there is excessive yang on the skin. This could be related to a meridian and appear only along that meridian, or it could appear all over the body – thus making it a Lung problem. It is more common in darker-skinned patients and those exposed to the sun.

Unfortunately, I do not know how to make these areas disappear. If, however, the intention is to reduce the appearance of these areas, then it helps to cool the skin – this involves sedating the yang of the meridian that manifests the pigmentation or sedating the Lung yang if the patches are in many areas.

- When sedating the yang meridians, one could sedate directly – sedate pigmentation on the maxillary area (Stomach channel) with St 45 sedation.

- When sedating the yang of a yin meridian, one should sedate it indirectly, over the coupled yang meridian – sedate Lung yang by sedating LI 2.

One other simple suggestion which I have found to be very useful is for the patient to follow at home:

1. Boil full-fat milk, until the skin begins to form. Skim off the skin and collect it in a saucer. Let it cool in a refrigerator, then apply it to the hyperpigmented area (and on the areas prone to pigmentation). Wash off after 20 minutes. Using a fresh preparation each time, repeat this treatment two or three times a week.

2. Another treatment is to slice potatoes thinly and leave the slices in a pile exposed to the air until they get a bit soggy. Then place these slices on the hyperpigmented area and leave for 15 minutes. Remove the potatoes and clean the skin.

CHAPTER 7

COSMETIC ACUPUNCTURE

CHAPTER CONTENTS

I bet you couldn't wait to reach this point in the book! Most readers would have been more interested in this part of the book than the dermatology part. But there is a very good reason why this is the last section: if one does not understand the skin and the connective tissue, if one cannot treat skin diseases with good results, then it is not possible for one to obtain good results with cosmetic acupuncture. One needs some experience with day-to-day problems of the skin and the rest of the body before dealing with enhancing beauty and delaying ageing. *Cosmetic acupuncture is primarily about health – not about beauty.*

All therapists believe that they have magical powers in their hands when they get to learn cosmetic acupuncture. They forget that these magical powers were in their hands to begin with when they trained in the theory and practice of traditional Chinese medicine. This book, my small experience, only puts this knowledge together for you. This is why, I am sure, you keep recognizing many little facts and observations I make as we go along.

In this chapter, we will discuss common cosmetic problems and their treatment.

A TYPICAL COSMETIC FACE LIFTING TREATMENT

- The patient is ushered into the treatment room. The patient is given a glass of water and advised to sip this occasionally (drinking little and often is necessary for the treatment to work but it is better not drink too much, so as to avoid having to interrupt treatment for the patient to go to the toilet). Advise the patient to have a light dinner before 7 p.m. on the evening before treatment. No coffee or tea is permitted before treatment. If the face is to be treated locally, then all make-up should be removed.

- The patient has a short chat with the therapist (unless it is their initial consultation) and then treatment begins.

- If there is any face lifting or wrinkle needling to be done, local anaesthetic cream will be applied to these areas at this stage. I use Emla local anaesthetic cream. The therapist should take care not to get Emla cream on his or her fingers, as this will result in loss of sensitivity in manipulating the needle.

- The patient now usually lies down and undergoes a normal body acupuncture treatment with appropriate energy-balancing points, and moxibustion where necessary. This takes 20 minutes.

- The body needles are removed, and the patient is asked to sit upright on a comfortable armchair – but not a recliner – so that gravity can be worked against.

- The needles are then applied on the face for the face lifting or wrinkle treatment or both. Needles are left *in situ* for 30 minutes, and manipulated every 10 minutes.

- At the end of 30 minutes, we prepare to remove the needles. The patient holds an open tube of arnica cream, while each needle is manipulated finally and removed slowly. If there is any bleeding at this point, arnica cream is applied to the area and pressure applied.

- Once the needles are all removed, the patient should avoid going out in the heat for about 10 minutes in case of delayed bruising. They are then free to do as they please.

Not all cosmetic treatments are like this. But face lifting is somewhat special.

Let us move on to the common problems and the energy imbalances. If you would like a quick reference, you can refer to Table 7.1 at the end of this chapter. Some of the following conditions respond very well to local treatment, together with the body treatment. For each problem I will include some or all of the following:

1. Body acupuncture treatment (energy-balancing points) – treating the cause of the problem.

2. Special local therapy – treating the area where the problem manifests.

3. What the patient can do at home to help treatment and extend the period of effect.

7.1 THIN, WRINKLY SKIN

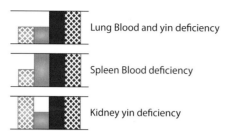

Lung Blood and yin deficiency

Spleen Blood deficiency

Kidney yin deficiency

- Start by applying oil on the area to be worked with. I use a warming oil such as 'Red oil' or St John's Wort oil.

The best way to describe this is as 'smoker's skin'. The skin is prematurely aged, perhaps also with thin brows and less head hair. This is more common in thin patients and smokers. I have also seen this in people following a severe low-fat diet. The skin is poorly nourished and is very dry.

- As the Lung gets its nutrition from its mother organ, the Spleen, it is necessary to ensure there is enough nutrition for the Spleen itself. The Spleen needs to be tonified with food and needles. Believe it or not, the best way to tonify Spleen Blood (nutrition) is by consuming some oily and fatty foods. The safe choice is to drink a tub (1/4 l) of buttermilk per day ('a buttermilk a day keeps the wrinkles away') This makes the skin thicker and more full. Considering the possibility that the Spleen could get damp easily, it would be better to drink the buttermilk during mid-morning, around 10.30 a.m.

- The next point is to take care of the moisture. The Kidneys irrigate the whole body with water. When the Kidneys are yin deficient (because the patient is in menopause, or drinks too many diuretic drinks such as coffee, tea and alcohol, or has excessive heat in the body that uses up thin fluids), then the Kidneys draw water from the mother organ, the Lung, thus making the Lungs yin deficient. It is the patient's responsibility, therefore, to drink water regularly and throughout the day, and avoid heat-producing foods and diuretic drinks in excess.

- If the patient is a smoker there is nothing we can do that would work for them.

- If these patients are not too old (under 65), there is hope for this problem. The good news is that no local needling is involved.

7.1.1 Body acupuncture treatment

To tonify Lung yin and Blood

- Lu 1 – Front-mu point – cools the skin.

- Lu 9 – tonification point – receives energy from the mother organ, the Spleen.

- Ren 17 – given in the direction to the face – the master point for the respiratory organs and skin.

- Humidify the air around by using a water spray, potted plants or humidifier.

For tonifying Spleen Blood and nutrition

- Sp 3 – own-element point, tonifies the yin.

- Drink a quarter-litre tub of buttermilk daily; use vegetable oil as a marinade for salad and meat.

- Eat more protein and grains and slow-cooked chicken soup.

For tonifying Kidney yin

- K 10.

- Drink water throughout the day.

- Add some salt to the diet unless there is a medical reason for not doing so. This will help retain water in the body.

- Avoid heat-producing foods and diuretic drinks.

All the points and suggestions above should be used simultaneously. The treatment is given twice weekly for 2 weeks and continued once weekly for six more weeks, or longer in severe cases.

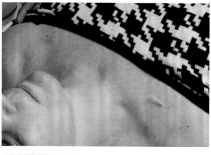
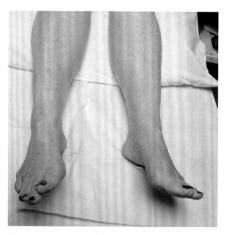
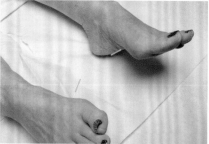
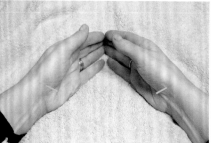
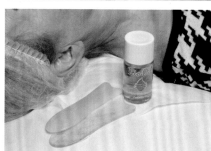

7.1.2 Special local therapy

- Gua Sha technique.

- Laser with hyaluronic acid preparation.

- Individual fine-line needling.

These therapies are described below.

GUA SHA TECHNIQUE

- Use a Gua Sha instrument or a thin saucer or Chinese soup spoon, and rub the area in upward and outward motions. Work on one side of the face or body until the skin becomes red and full, then proceed to the other side. It takes 2–3 minutes to work on an area – so ensure that you take a large enough area for that amount of time. Do not continue to rub an area if red petechiae start to appear. We do not want this in cosmetic treatments.

- Gua Sha treatment is done only once a week. Laser or fine-line needling could be done if the patient comes for a second treatment in the same week.

- Gua Sha gives an immediate 'filled' look. The skin has a red glow after the treatment, but this settles before the next day. Direct exposure to sunlight should be avoided when there is redness.

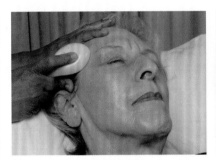 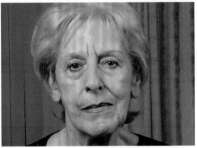

A   B

Figure 7.1 (A) Gua Sha treatment of face. Treatment should stop if red spots appear; (B) after Gua Sha on one side; the other side has not been treated.

Use some oil on the skin surface that you are about to treat. I use red oil (St John's wort oil), which is suitable for almost all patients. If the patient has very thin and sensitive skin, they may react to this oil with some red wheals, especially if they go in the sun after treatment. It would be better to use ordinary baby oil on these patients. Also, I find Bio Oil to be extremely good. It is important that no cooling oils, such as oils with mint, aloe vera or tea tree oil, are used with this treatment.

Dry your hands after applying the oil so that they are not slippery. Use a Gua Sha instrument (I prefer the fish-shaped one).

Gua Sha on the face involves three procedures:

- Cutting.
- Smoothing.
- Lifting.

Cutting

Stretch on both sides across the wrinkles with your fingers so that they look flattened. Holding the Gua Sha instrument with the sharp side vertical, cut or scratch the wrinkles at right angles.

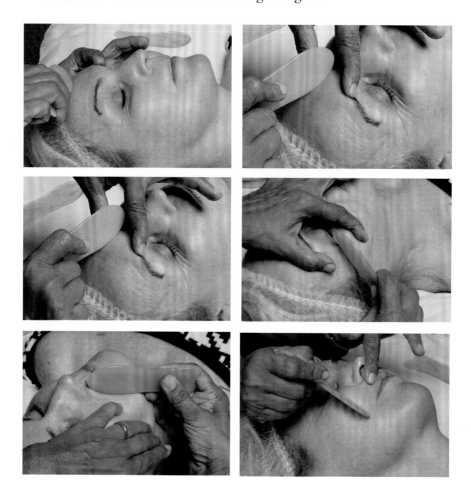

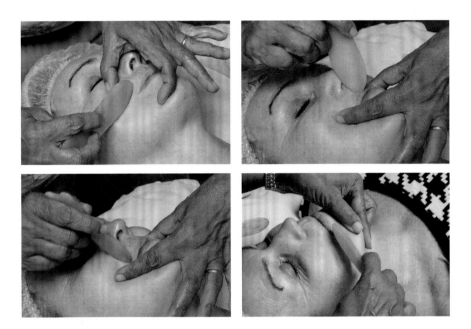

Do this several times in both upwards and downwards directions. This is done in order to create minute injuries in the depths of the wrinkles, therefore it is important that it is done in the deepest part of the wrinkles. The cutting is done on the forehead, around the eyes, between the brows, at the sides of the mouth, and anywhere else fine wrinkles can be found on the face and neck.

Smoothing

After cutting or scratching the wrinkles, smooth the skin with the flat part of the Gua Sha instrument. You should always do this in an upwards and outwards direction from the midline of the face.

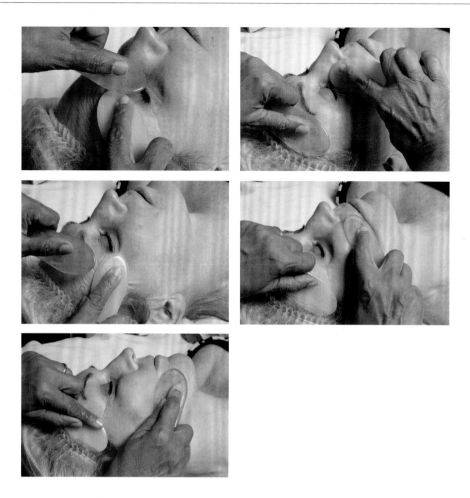

This part of the procedure takes the longest time, including lymphatic drainage, extending to the neck and jawline. This will produce the 'wow' effect, so time should be taken until you are satisfied with the result.

Lifting

As the smoothing has been done in a lifting direction, the 'lifting strokes' have already begun. But, as an additional step, you could do more. For instance, when going over the upper eyelid, you could slow down and, with the patient's eyes closed, use the flat of the Gua Sha stick to prise open the eyelid – thus creating an 'open-eyed' look.

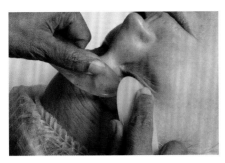
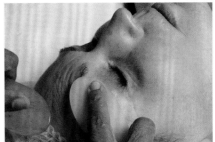
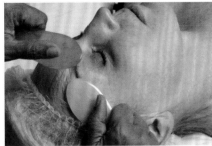

The same could be done on the upper lip. After smoothing the small wrinkles above the upper lip, use the flat of the Gua Sha stick to turn the upper lip upwards several times, and this creates a lifting effect on the upper lip.

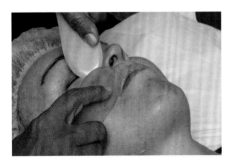

Jaw defining should be done at this time. Using the tail of the fish stick, define the jawline and finish with five strokes of lymph drainage.

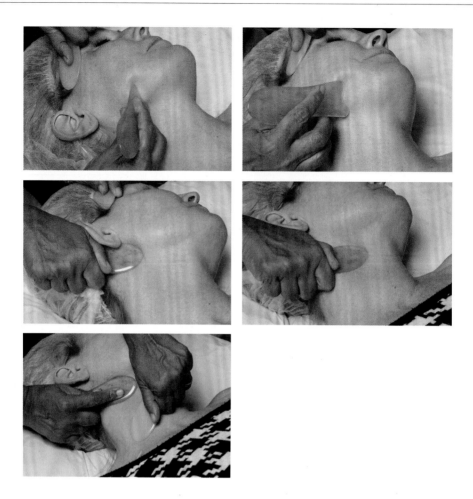

As a final touch, take two Gua Sha sticks (preferably jade sticks, as they will cool down the skin) and use both in the lifting direction quite firmly and quickly, in order to do the lifting.

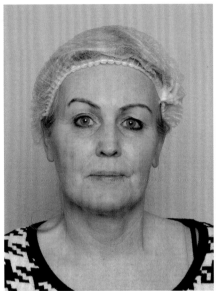

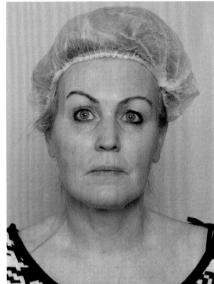

BEFORE   AFTER

If you wish to use any skin rejuvenation creams, this should be done at the end of the Gua Sha session. I would suggest Hyaluronic acid application in extremely dry skin with hyperpigmentation, and collagen gel for general revitalization. Don't use Hyaluronic acid on puffy or swollen eyelids, as this will cause worsening of the situation.

Laser treatment for skin rejuvenation is the last possible addition to this treatment. You could carry out 15 minutes of polylaser derma at the end of the session.

SKIN REJUVENATION THERAPY WITH HYALURONIC ACID AND POLYLASER DERMA

- The patient should remove all make-up the night before.
- Clean skin thoroughly. This treatment is expensive, and works on the basis of the hyaluronic acid being absorbed into the skin.
- Use a wet or dry warming pad to warm the area to be worked on.
- Drop the bottle of hyaluronic acid into a bowl of very hot water to loosen the gel.
- Using a syringe, draw out the required amount of hyaluronic acid, and apply to the skin to be worked on.
- Perform a massage on the skin until all the gel has been absorbed.
- Seal the gel in by adding few drops of water at the end of massage.
- Irradiate the area with Polylaser Derma for approximately 10–15 minutes over an area of 15 cm^2.
- It is important for both patient and therapist to wear protective glasses.
- Treatment is performed generally once a week in the first 2 weeks and then once or twice a month.
- The patient leaves the clinic with glowing skin. This therapy not only rejuvenates the skin, but delays skin ageing.

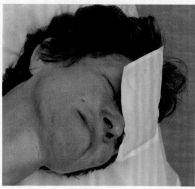 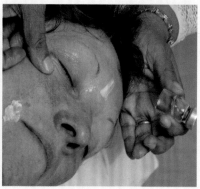

A   B

Figure 7.2 Laser therapy for thin, wrinkly skin. (A) Place warm pack on the area to be treated; (B) apply and massage the hyaluronic acid before laser treatment

FINE WRINKLE TREATMENT WITH NEEDLES

- The needles are removed after 30 minutes.
- The needles are twirled every 10 minutes.
- Twirl the needles around in two full circles (720°) in a clockwise direction. This is the best manipulation for cell rejuvenation.
- Insert needles subcutaneously into the wrinkle, needling the entire wrinkle with as many needles as it takes. On the face, I use 15 mm SEIRIN® needles. Needle one wrinkle in one direction.
- This treatment is given with body acupuncture. So it would be good to apply some local anaesthetic cream (I use Emla cream) on the lines as soon as the patient comes in. It takes about 20–30 minutes to numb the area. This is a treatment for individual fine but stubborn lines around the eyes, mouth, forehead, etc. (Figure 7.3). There is stronger treatment for deep lines.

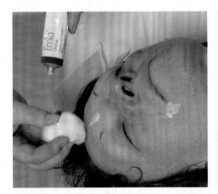
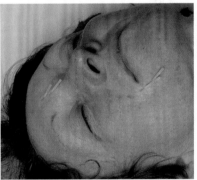

A   B

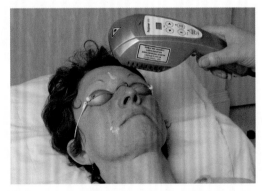

C

Figure 7.3 Fine wrinkle needling. (A) Apply local anaesthetic cream on wrinkle; (B) needle subcutaneously through wrinkle and rotate needle 720 ° clockwise; (C) use Polylaser Derma on treated wrinkle to expedite building of collagen (alpha frequency).

7.1.3 What the patient can do at home
Egg mask on face

- Beat a whole egg.

- Paint it onto the face and neck.

- Repeat after 10 minutes.

- After the second application, leave it to dry for 20 minutes.

- Wash off.

- Repeat once or twice a week.

Mung dhall mask on face

This is suitable for patients willing to put in a little more effort.

- Soak green mung dhall overnight in water.

- Grind it in a wet grinder.

- Apply on slightly wet skin.

- Remove the dhall paste after 30 minutes.

- Wash off.

- Repeat once a week.

These treatments give protein directly to the skin. It would also help if the patient uses a rich moisturizing cream on the face and neck skin both in the morning and evening.

7.2 HANGING, PUFFY SKIN

 Spleen Qi deficiency

This is the sagging that occurs in early middle age, first in parts of the body that are not readily visible, but later on in the face. This loss of firmness is caused by loose connective tissue, which should hold our skin firmly to the muscle below (Figure 7.4), which, in turn, is caused by Spleen Qi deficiency. This gets worse as the patient gets older and also (1) *heavier*, when there is more skin and fat to attach to the muscle, or (2) *thinner*, when the Spleen also becomes Blood deficient, making the connective tissue weaker.

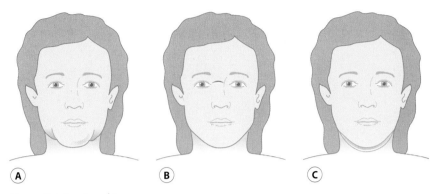

Figure 7.4 Sagging skin

One cannot firm up connective tissue by working out, but exercise for muscle toning would help to an extent and should be encouraged. Local plum-blossom tapping is a very effective method to treat sagging and puffy or loose skin. Cosmetic face lifting is the treatment of choice here.

The body treatment for this problem is to tonify the Spleen Qi. This can be done directly by tonifying the yang aspect of the Spleen, and, very importantly, by eating a proper diet. This is what would retain the results of the face lifting treatment.

Other products for skin rejuvenation

Hyaluronic acid is not suitable for patients who have swollen eyelids or oedema on the face, or for patients with chronic sinusitis with dampness and oedema around the sinuses. Also, when the skin is uneven and has many different coloured areas of pigmentation, there is a better product one could use. This product is called collagen gel (platinum). it is made of fish skin and is not a synthetic product. One should use this each morning, on a clean, wet face, and use a moisturizer over it. If make-up is to be applied, this should be applied over the moisturizer.

In the evenings, the skin should cleansed thoroughly, and a light night cream used before bed.

Using collagen gel is an excellent maintenance between treatment sessions. It smooths, nourishes and rejuvenates the skin.

7.2.1 Body acupuncture treatment

FOR TONIFYING SPLEEN YANG AND QI

- Sp 1 – the wood point and grandmother point of the Spleen tonifies the Spleen yang. This point could be warmed with a moxa cigar for a stronger effect. If the patient has gastritis or other heat problems of the Stomach, then needling this point would be better than moxa.

- UB 20 – Back-Shu point of the Spleen – improves function (Qi).

- St 36 – as the Spleen is a yin organ and we are trying to improve the yang, this point which improves the Stomach yang would indirectly tonify the Spleen yang as well.

- *The basic difference between Spleen Qi and yang is that yang causes warming, and Qi does not necessarily.* When treating to tone connective tissue we mainly need to tonify the Spleen Qi, because to tone or firm is a function. But if the patient who is to be given this firming treatment has very cold extremities most of the time and gets Stomach pain if eating or drinking anything cold, then they probably have both Qi and yang deficiency of the Spleen and Stomach. If the yang is deficient, it is quite difficult to improve only the function,[1] as yang or warmth activates the function and the cold retards it. Here it is necessary to tonify the yang as well as the Qi. So moxa should be used on more points – Sp 1, Ren 12, St 36, and warm and cooked food should be eaten – raw and cold meals should be avoided.

- The correct diet to strengthen the Spleen Qi is therefore also cooked and warm food and drink – eating more protein, unrefined carbohydrates and cooked vegetables and fruits. Fatty foods should be avoided, as should refined sugars and carbohydrates and raw, cold food and drinks – less should be eaten but more often so as not to overtire the Spleen. It is also very important to eat less and early in the evenings, so as to avoid eating at the Stomach

---

1   The reverse is not true. There may be heat in the Stomach (e.g. gastritis) or Spleen (e.g. pancreatitis, parotitis or lymph gland inflammation), but this pathogenic heat will not activate the function of the Spleen or Stomach. In fact, this pathogenic heat will even inhibit the normal function of the organ. When treating to tonify the Qi in such cases, moxa or heat introducing needle technique should not be used as these may increase the yang.

and Spleen's lowest function time according to our organ clock –
between 7.00 p.m. and 11.00 p.m.

7.2.2 Special local therapy

- Cosmetic face lifting – face, neck, breast.

- Plum-blossom tapping to firm connective tissue – chin, abdomen,
  eyelids.

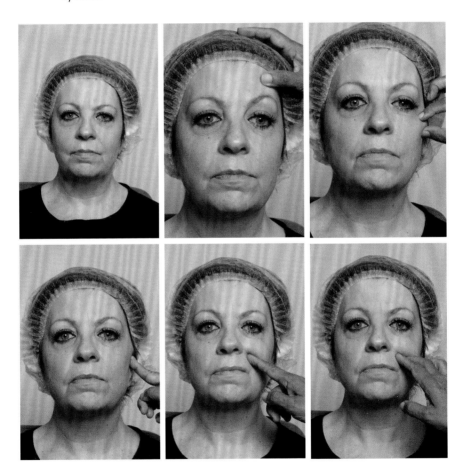

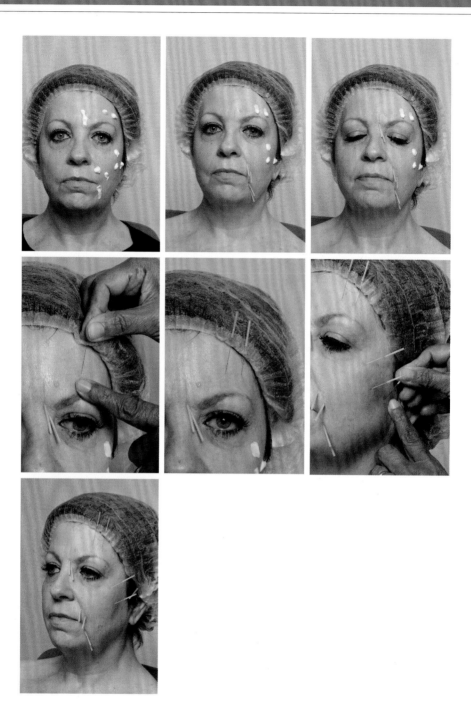

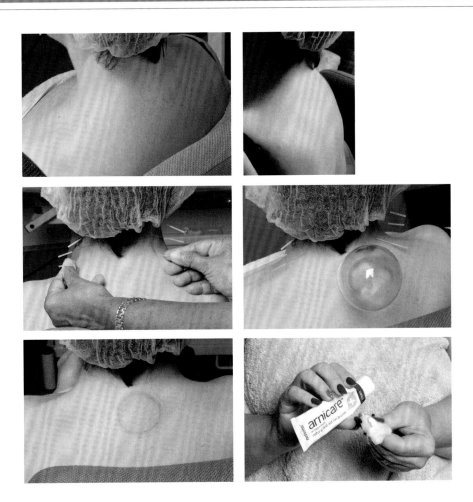

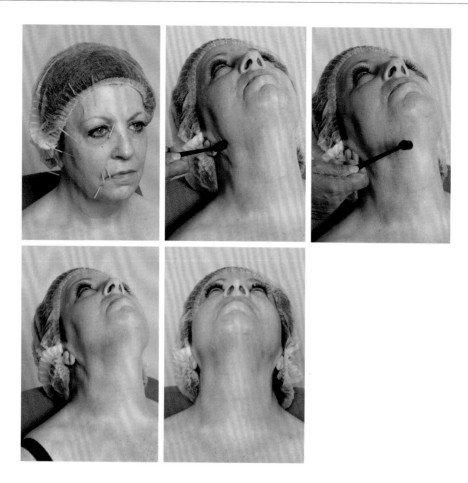

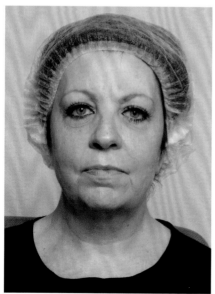

BEFORE

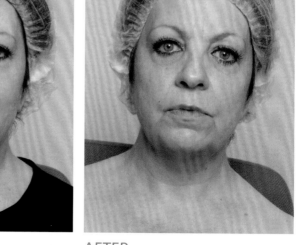

AFTER

COSMETIC FACE LIFTING

- As soon as the patient enters the surgery local anaesthetic cream should be applied to the areas where the face and neck needles will go in. These creams take approximately 20–30 minutes to work. Use cotton wool to apply the anaesthetic cream, so your fingers are not numbed. Some patients prefer not to have an anaesthetic – it is up to them to decide.

- The patient lies down and is needled in the body acupuncture points for energy balancing. Make sure that the room is not overheated, so as not to cause later bleeding.

- After 20 minutes, the body needles come off, the patient sits up on a comfortable straight armed chair (not a recliner!) and is ready for the lifting points.

- The points are given at an angle of 45° to the midline, from the side. The points are not necessarily acupuncture points, but have to be judged initially by lifting the skin with the hands, to see if it makes a difference (Figure 7.5C).

- All needles should have the muscle as the final place of entry.

- After all needles have been inserted, the needles are tightened, with the thumb twirled in the upward and outward direction to the midline (Figure 7.5), and always in one direction only.

- You can observe the lifting effect within minutes! If only one side of the face is treated (as it often is for demonstration purposes), the effect is very clear to see.

- The needles should be reinforced every 10 minutes after insertion. This means that they are pushed slightly deeper, and the thumb twirled to the midline again.

- At the end of 30 minutes, the needles should be tightened for the last time and then removed.

- When removing the needles, they should not be twirled or loosened. The knot that was created in the depth should be retained, and the needle should be pulled out very slowly as the therapist's finger remains pressed on this knot.

- This is a tense moment as there is possibility of a haematoma, which a cosmetic patient will not appreciate. So keep an open tube of Arnica cream ready at hand (usually in the patient's hand). If there is a haematoma, press immediately on the point with the cream.

- The patient should not go into the sun for 10 minutes following extraction of the needles, as the blood vessels could dilate and delayed bleeding may occur.

- Cosmetic face lifting can be performed twice weekly initially, for 1–3 weeks. The chances of bleeding increase then, so it would be better to do one session per week thereafter.

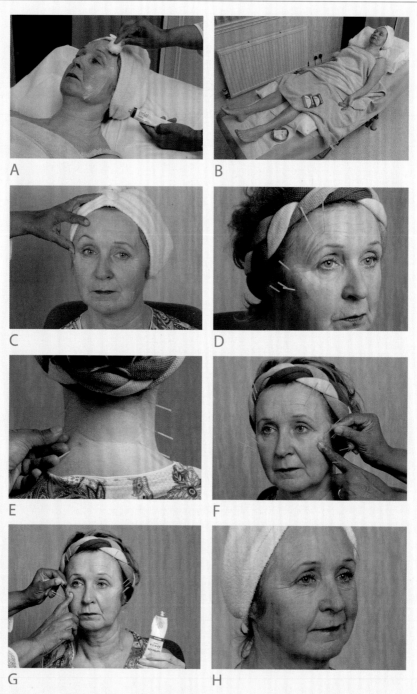

Figure 7.5 Cosmetic face lift. (A) Applying local anaesthetic; (B) lying down for body acupuncture; (C) judging where lifting should be done; (D) seven lifting needles from forehead to cheek; (E) firming the neck from the back; (F) needle manipulation to cause firming – note the upward and outward twirling of the thumb; (G) needles removed without twirling, while the knot is held firmly under the finger; (H) after treatment.

PLUM-BLOSSOM TAPPING FOR PUFFY EYELIDS

- The patient's eyes are closed. Pull the corner of the eye outwards to give it some tension.
- Tap with hammer, always clockwise to the therapist (both eyes) around the eye. Tapping should be very light.
- Seven circles make one treatment; eight to ten sessions make a course.

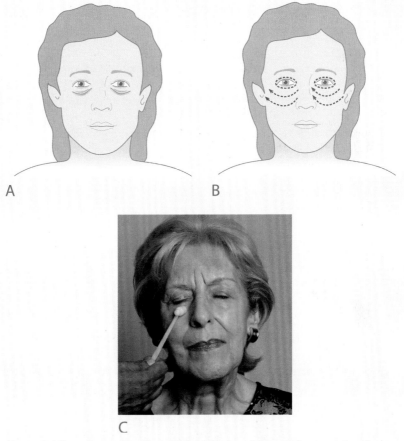

Figure 7.6 Treatment of puffy eyelids with plum-blossom hammer tapping

PLUM-BLOSSOM TAPPING FOR FIRMING THE CHIN

This is ideally done with the patient sitting up, though it is hard on the practitioner's back as you have to bend to the patient's chin level. It is excellent in improving a hanging chin following weight loss or when the patient has sagging in this area.

- Imagine a triangle drawn between point SI 17, the Adam's apple and the tip of the chin.
- Tap with plum-blossom needle from the chin towards point SI 17, then in lines from the wider part of the triangle to the narrow part (Figure 7.7), until there is a red skin reaction.
- Repeat on the other side of the chin.
- This treatment is also good to prevent overeating.
- It can be repeated each time with face lifting therapy.

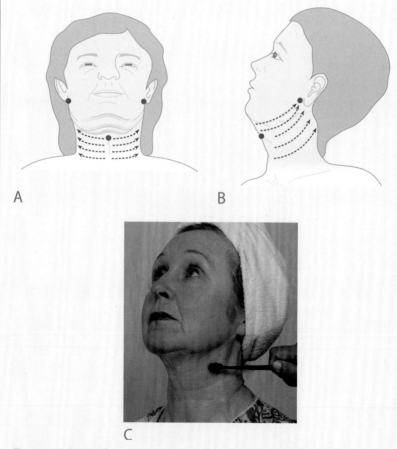

Figure 7.7 (A, B) Plum-blossom tapping of chin, for lifting; (C) plum-blossom tapping for firming the chin

PLUM-BLOSSOM TAPPING FOR FIRMING THE ABDOMEN

This treatment is excellent in patients who want to restore firmness to their skin while losing weight or after childbirth. It is not really helpful for obese patients.

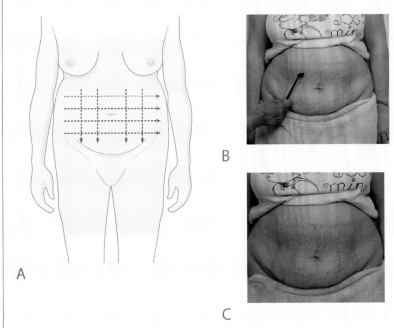

Figure 7.8 Plum-blossom tapping for abdomen lifting

- The patient should stand against a wall for stability. It would help if they stood on a higher step or stage, as the therapist has to bend to work at the abdomen level of the patient.

- The plum-blossom tapping is always from the left to the right of the abdomen along horizontal lines, and from up to down along vertical lines.

- Choose two lines left of the navel and two on the right for the vertical lines; two above and two below the navel for the horizontal lines. Each line should be tapped until a red skin reaction forms – roughly 10 to 15 times. The tapping should be light enough so as not to cause bleeding.

- When all lines are tapped, the red reaction will spread and the lines will widen.

- Treatment is done twice weekly for 2 weeks; then once weekly for a further 4 weeks. A firming effect can be seen after one treatment.

BREAST LIFTING WITH NEEDLES

In the early days of women's liberation, when women often went without a bra, the result was often sagging breasts, even in young women who had never given birth. The problem is worse in mothers. A combination of Spleen Qi deficiency causing loose connective tissue and heavy breasts is sure to cause sagging. As long as the breasts are not too large and heavy, this treatment should help.

- The body acupuncture should include points UB 15, UB 17 and UB 20.
- The patient should sit in a high chair after body acupuncture.
- Insert needles (Figure 7.9) in a fan-like design from the side of the breast to the top, all needles facing the nipple. The needles should enter the pectoral muscle, and not the breast tissue.
- Once all needles are inserted, the twisting-firming technique for lifting (with thumb twisting in the upwards and outwards direction away from the midline) should be employed.
- The needles should be reinforced every 10 minutes.
- At the end of 30 minutes, the needles should be strengthened one last time, and then removed slowly, without any twirling, so as to retain the tension at the point.
- Treatment can be repeated twice weekly for four times; then once a week for another four sessions.

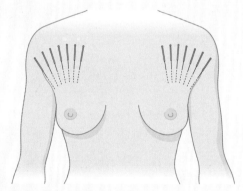

Figure 7.9 Breast lifting with needles

7.2.3 What the patient can do at home

It is very important that patients follow a proper diet at home. When they eat badly, the effects can be seen on their face the very next morning.

They should avoid damp-producing foods such as fatty foods, fatty milk products, fried foods, refined carbohydrates and sugars, alcohol, and cold and raw foods.

Although oily foods are not recommended, it is acceptable to use vegetable oil as a marinade or a dressing for cooked vegetables. It is heated oil that is damp producing.

Although unrefined carbohydrates and sugars are permitted, it is preferable to reduce consumption of any carbohydrates. This helps in firming the connective tissue.

Finally, all foods eaten after 6.00 p.m. will reduce the Spleen Qi, and so the patient should try hard to avoid this. A clear soup made from tomatoes, mushrooms, leafy vegetables – onions, leeks, spinach, cabbage, celery, and parsley – and containing a small piece of meat or fish for flavour can be taken in any quantity.

It is important that the patient drinks warm water and fluids, and eats warm food. Consumption of cold food and drinks will cool the Spleen and Stomach yang, which in turn will inhibit the functional Qi and the tone of the connective tissue.

7.3 SWOLLEN FACE

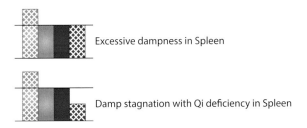

Excessive dampness in Spleen

Damp stagnation with Qi deficiency in Spleen

Generally speaking, a swollen face is just part of a bigger picture. This could be oedema in the whole body such as in Kidney failure or just poor function of the Kidneys, or it could be part of a peripheral oedema, involving Spleen Qi deficiency. It is up to the therapist to find out if it is an elimination or a circulation problem.

7.3.1 Body acupuncture treatment

- If it is an *elimination* problem, the urine will become reduced and there may be proteinuria. Kidney oedema is less of a problem in the mornings on waking, but gradually worsens during the day and is at its worst in the evenings. When Kidney function is deficient, urine output is best at night when the patient is lying down, and not as good during the day. It is unlikely that such a patient would request cosmetic therapies. However, points UB 23 with needle and cupping, K 3 and UB 58 Luo-connecting point are a good combination for improving urine output. Reducing salt intake will also help.

- It is more common for it to be a *circulation* problem. The Spleen is responsible for peripheral circulation of fluid. When the Spleen has excessive dampness (acute) or stagnation of dampness (chronic), then the face, lower arms and legs will become swollen. Spleen oedema is at its worst in the mornings on waking, because the patient has been dormant and there is insufficient Qi to circulate the fluid. The oedema improves during the activity of the day and is at its minimum in the late afternoon. This should respond well to point UB 20 with needle and cupping, and St 40 and Sp 9. The patient should avoid damp-producing foods such as fats, milk products, refined sugars and carbohydrates and late meals in the evenings.

7.3.2 What the patient can do at home

- Salt holds water – and so it is best to consume less under these circumstances. But salt baths, and a face towel soaked in warm salty water, wrung semi-dry and spread on the face for a few minutes, is good because it will help remove oedema from the face through osmosis.

7.4 SWOLLEN EYELIDS

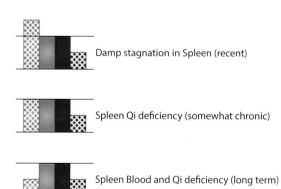

Damp stagnation in Spleen (recent)

Spleen Qi deficiency (somewhat chronic)

Spleen Blood and Qi deficiency (long term)

A whole swollen face indicates severe dampness, whereas swollen eyelids reflect a milder state of dampness. It is a symptom of Spleen Qi deficiency, and the quantity of dampness in the Spleen will depend on how long the symptoms have been present: the longer the oedema has been present, the lower the Spleen Blood will be. One function of Spleen Qi is to absorb nutrition from food and drink – and if the Spleen Qi has been deficient for a long time, then the absorbed nutrition for Blood-building will become gradually less, which causes Spleen Blood deficiency.

So when the Spleen Qi deficiency is relatively recent, the patient will appear well nourished or even adipose; when it becomes a chronic problem, the patient is moderately nourished; when it is very chronic, the patient is rather thin or malnourished. The peripheral oedema – on eyelids, hands and feet or on face, arms and legs – will be proportionate to this.

7.4.1 Body acupuncture treatment

- Spleen damp stagnation, relatively new state – UB 20, Sp 9, St 40, GB 20 and LI 4.

- Spleen Qi deficiency, chronic state – UB 20, St 36, Sp 1, GB 20 and LI 4.

- Spleen Blood and Qi deficiency – Liv 3, UB 20, Sp 3 and St 36, GB 20 and LI 4.

If the patient often has spotting between menstruation or bruises often, Sp 1 can be administered with moxa.

7.4.2 What the patient can do at home

In all three states, it is important to avoid damp foods. No local needling is advised. If the Spleen Qi is better, the stagnation will improve on its own. However, the patient can help by doing the treatment below at home.

- Dissolve two tablespoons of sea salt granules in a cup of water; thinly slice a cucumber and soak in the water in the refrigerator. Lying down, place the slices of cucumber around the eyes, with the eyes shut. Remove after 10 minutes. This can be done daily or whenever the oedema is severe.

7.5 DARK RINGS BELOW THE EYES

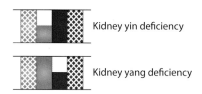

Kidney yin deficiency

Kidney yang deficiency

Grey or blue colour anywhere on the face or tongue is a sign of Kidney deficiency. Unfortunately, it does not tell us which aspect of the Kidney is weak. We have to rely on other information in order to find out what aspect is deficient, keeping in mind that both yin and yang could be weak in the Kidney.

7.5.1 Body acupuncture treatment

Kidney yin deficiency

There will be considerable dryness. The tongue can be dry and cracked and the skin will also be quite dry. The urine will be concentrated and low in volume; the stools can be hard and dark. There may be hot flushes and night sweating and the patient may feel energetic after rest and at nights but feel quite exhausted around midday.

- K 7 or K 10 (to tonify Kidney yin).

- GB 20 and LI 4 (for the eyes).

These symptoms will show us that the Kidney yin and water are quite low in the body. The patient needs to drink water regularly, eat watery foods and fruits, and points K 7 or K 10 will be suitable in this case, along with GB 20 and LI 4 for the eyes.

Resting the eye with a cooling gel pad intermittently, a good night's sleep beginning well before midnight and applying milk to the skin are what the patient can do to improve the situation. If treated early, this is successfully eliminated. A chronic problem may not be so easy to treat.

Kidney yang deficiency

- UB 23, K 3 (tonifies Kidney yang).

- UB 67 (tonifies Urinary Bladder yang and therefore, indirectly, Kidney yang).

As the Kidney function is low, there will be water retention. The face and even the eyelids can be swollen, as may the feet and ankles. Urination at night will be greater than that during the day, and the urine can be turbid. There may be initial stiffness and coldness in the joints, especially in the knees and back. The patient has energy problems when starting the day, but feels reasonable by midday. They might be timid, fearful people.

As these are symptoms of Kidney yang deficiency, it would be good to treat this with points UB 23, K 3 and UB 67, and encourage the patient to do regular exercise or sports, especially exercise involving the back (such as push-ups). Warmth is as good as any treatment, and exposure to cold should be avoided.

Red fish, the legs and feet of animals (chicken feet, pig trotters) and fish with bones (sardines, bait and shellfish) are all good sources of Kidney yang.

7.5.2 What the patient can do at home

Milk skin application

Boil milk in a pan until a skin forms on top. Remove this skin, and store it in the fridge. Apply thickly around the eyes; if too dry, wet with some cold milk. Wash off after 20 minutes.

Chickpea flour application

This idea was given to me by one of my patients! I have tried it and it works on hyperpigmentation in general.

Add a tablespoon of chickpea flour, half a teaspoon of turmeric, a little almond oil, a squeeze of lemon and yoghurt, and apply it to the hyperpigmented area. After 15 minutes, it can be washed off. Do not cleanse the area till the next day.

Hyaluronic acid application

Patients can use hyaluronic acid at home about twice a week. This has to be applied on very clean skin, which has been warmed and moistened. Apply the hyaluronic acid sparingly and massage it through the pigmented area, finishing with some drops of water or a light moisturizer at the end. Leave it overnight.

7.6 DULL SKIN

 Lung yang deficiency (also Kidney yang deficiency)

 Lung Qi deficiency (also Kidney Qi deficiency)

Youthful skin has a shine. It exudes life energy in the same way that the sun radiates light. This is what happens when the Lung Qi reaches the skin surface and when the Kidney gives life energy to all tissues of the body. But when the Lung Qi is too weak to rise to the skin, and if the Kidneys are weak in yang and Qi, then the skin will look dead. Make-up can improve the colour, but cannot bring life to the skin for more than a few moments – and the more make-up used to conceal the lifeless look, the worse the skin will become as the Qi gets blocked from rising to the surface.

7.6.1 Body acupuncture treatment

POINTS TO TONIFY LUNG YANG AND QI

- UB 13, Lu 10 and LI 11.

POINTS TO TONIFY KIDNEY YANG AND QI

- UB 23, K 3 and UB 67.

POINTS TO TONIFY BLOOD IF SKIN IS PALE

- UB 13, UB 15, Ren 14, Lu 1, Sp 10, UB 17 and GB 39.

7.6.2 Special local therapy

- Hyaluronic acid with Polylaser Derma for skin rejuvenation.

7.6.3 What the patient can do at home

- In winter, it would help to take a sauna or Turkish bath once a week.

- Have alternating hot and cold showers.

- Consume hot soups containing ginger root.

- Take regular exercise and participate in sports in order to encourage sweating.

7.7 DULL, LIFELESS HAIR

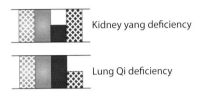

Kidney yang deficiency

Lung Qi deficiency

This is another symptom of Qi and life energy not reaching the skin and roots of the head hair. As head hair is directly nourished by the Kidney, this is first a Kidney yang deficiency; and as the scalp is an extension of the facial skin, this is also a Lung Qi deficiency. We have already discussed loss of hair and damaged hair. Now we are concentrating only on the appearance of the hair – hair that is very oily and heavy or is dirty and sticky and needs to be washed.

7.7.1 Body acupuncture treatment

To tonify Kidney yang

- UB 23, K 3 and UB 67.

To tonify Lung Qi

- UB 13, Lu 10 and LI 11.

To tonify Blood (when appropriate)

- Ren 14, UB 15, Lu 1, UB 13, Sp 10, UB 17 and GB 39.

These points could be added for dull eyes

- GB 20, UB 10 and LI 4.

7.7.2 What the patient can do at home

The best way to bring yang and Qi to an area of the body is to bring Blood flow to that area (just as the quickest way to cool a hot area is to bleed the area). In order to help the hair to become shiny and full of life and bounce, the quick and effective way is to bring Blood flow to the head. And how does one do this? Well, we could ask our patient to do a 10-minute head stand! Not very practical. Another option is for them to lie on a bed at home and hang their head forward, below the bed level. This is a comfortable position and it can be maintained for 10 minutes daily. This will bring shine and bounce to the hair within a few days! What's more, this is an excellent therapy against premature greying of head hair.

Many patients wash their hair daily and use volumizing agents and a hairdryer on a very hot setting to create the appearance of a head of shiny, bouncy hair. If one does this on a regular basis, this injures the hair and even causes loss of hair. A good vitamin product such as Pantovigar – N® (or any product containing thiamine nitrate, calcium pantothenate, cystine or keratin) will help to nourish the hair from within. Some olive oil or coconut oil can be used to massage into the scalp 20 minutes before washing, and the head kept warm with a hot towel wrap. Hair should be washed no more than twice weekly.

7.8 DRY HAIR WITH DANDRUFF

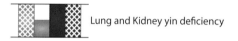 Lung and Kidney yin deficiency

Dry hair is another symptom of dry skin and scalp and also causes dandruff. Patients can help themselves by massaging olive oil or coconut oil into the scalp once a week and leaving it on overnight or for at least 30 minutes, with a hot towel wrapped around the head, then washing it off as usual. Drinking more water and humidifying the rooms will also help. Patients sometimes wash their hair too often in an attempt to get rid of the dandruff – it is better to brush the hair vigorously on a daily basis but to wash only twice a week to preserve the natural oils. Using hairspray to hold a style in place should be avoided as much as possible.

7.8.1 Body acupuncture treatment

POINTS TO TONIFY LUNG YIN

- Lu 1, Ren 17, Lu 9.

POINTS TO TONIFY KIDNEY YIN

- K 7 alternated with K 10, Ren 3, Sp 6.

These points can be used together, initially twice weekly, and later once a week. No local treatment is needed.

7.9 DEEP WRINKLES

Deep wrinkles are most common on the forehead and at the corners of the lips or eyes; the nasolabial groove can also be very deep in places sometimes. Wrinkles are mostly caused by facial movements such as constantly frowning or raising the brows. Patients should be made aware of this, and any underlying reason – for example, screwing up the eyes because eyesight is poor – should be corrected.

The good news is that a deep wrinkle can be treated reasonably well by combining cosmetic face lift with a local treatment for the wrinkle. The face lift will lift the skin away from the wrinkle and reduce the weight on it. The local treatment attempts to create a scar to make the wrinkle less obvious.

7.9.1 Special local therapy

This is a one-off treatment for one wrinkle.

- Apply local anaesthetic and leave for 20 minutes.

- Use a thick (No. 1) hypodermic needle for injection.

- Turning the needle with the cutting edge facing upwards (Figure 7.10), prick the skin and lift up the epithelium. The needle tip should be pointing towards the wrinkle and not at right angles to it.

- Do this along the wrinkle, each spot adjoining the other, so that a wrinkle as long as 1 cm will have at least 10 punctures.

- There will be bleeding and you must press and clean the skin so you can continue to see what you are doing.

- When the whole wrinkle has been punctured, go back to make sure the skin is broken along the line without interruption.

- Use the Polylaser Derma on the scar for 10 minutes, which will reduce healing time by half. If you do not have a laser, then leave the wound open and untreated.

- When the wound heals, the wrinkle will lose depth and become firm, and it will therefore become more difficult to see. This will take about 3 weeks.

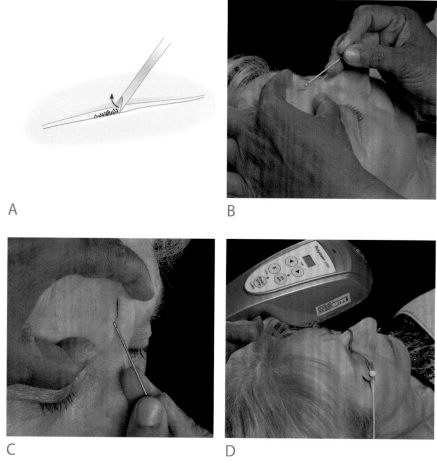

A

B

C

D

Figure 7.10 (A, B, C) Deep-wrinkle needling with hypodermic needle; (D) laser treatment after the wrinkle has been needled to expedite healing

7.9.2 What the patient can do at home

An egg or mung dhall face pack can be applied to the skin (see page 182). These should not be used until the wrinkle has healed completely.

7.10 CELLULITE

 Stagnation of damp and fat on Spleen and affected meridian

Cellulite usually begins around the hips and thighs and mostly along the yang meridians. The starting point is often the Gall Bladder, the lesser yang meridian, perhaps because the Qi in the Gall Bladder is less than in the other yang meridians. Cellulite describes dimpling of the skin, caused by the protrusion of subcutaneous fat into the dermis, creating an undulating junction between the skin and the subcutaneous adipose tissue.

The Spleen nourishes muscle and fat and the function of the Spleen is to distribute fatty tissue evenly through the body, especially in the periphery. In the case of cellulite, the fat distribution is affected, and fatty tissue seems to stagnate without flow in certain parts of the body. So, on the one hand there is excess fat, and on the other there is poor circulation of it. This creates the picture of imbalance described above.

However, there is also a problem in the meridian along which this problem occurs – which could be the Gall Bladder but may also be the Urinary Bladder or even the Stomach, depending on the patient. So both the Spleen and the affected meridians need to be balanced.

7.10.1 Body acupuncture treatment

Example – cellulite on the lateral side of thighs (Figures 7.11 and 7.12).

- Gall Bladder – UB 19 (Back-Shu point), GB 37 (Luo point).

- Spleen – UB 20 (Back-Shu point), St 40 (Luo point).

- Local needles and moving cup massage.
- Two sessions per week, eight to ten sessions in total.

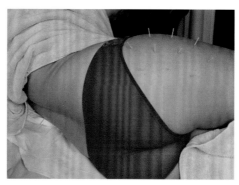

Figure 7.11 Local needling for cellulite

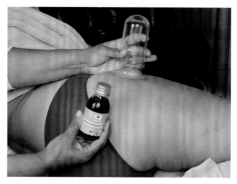

Figure 7.12 Cupping massage for cellulite

This treatment principle can be used in every affected meridian. For example, for the Bladder meridian – one could use UB 28 (the Back-Shu point, to improve the function) and UB 58 (the Luo-connecting point of the yang meridian, to tonify the yang and reduce the yin aspect).

Local treatment is very effective if performed well. Patients sometimes want to rush through local treatment because cupping massage is not very pleasant – it is important to persuade them to be patient.

7.10.2 Special local therapy

If the affected area is on the side along the Gall Bladder meridian, this treatment should be done in two halves, with the patient lying on one side first and having all the needles and cupping; then turning onto the other side and having the same treatment.

- Lying on the side, points on the body – UB 18, UB 20, St 40, GB 37.

- At the same time, about 10 to 15 local needles in the area of the cellulite (15–20 cm needles of 0.20 mm gauge) are inserted perpendicularly and completely, at about 3 cm distance from each other.

- Both body needles and local needles are left *in situ* for 20 minutes.

- After all the needles are removed, apply St John's wort oil sparingly on the area of cellulite. Do not overdo this, as it will reduce friction for the massage.

- Place a large cup (for a special cellulite cup, see Figure 7.12) at the lower end of the thigh using fire to create a vacuum, and slide the cup up and down along the area until the skin becomes quite red. This procedure is quite uncomfortable for the patient and, if very sore, the vacuum could be reduced. The massage takes about 1 minute.

- The patient may remark that the legs feel very light after the treatment.

7.10.3 What the patient can do at home

As cellulite is a stagnation of fatty tissue, the patient can do many things at home to prevent its formation and to improve circulation.

- Foods that create fat tissue in the body are fatty foods, fatty milk products (low-fat milk products can be consumed in moderation), refined carbohydrates and sugars (though unrefined carbohydrates, fruit, sugar and honey are fine). These foods should be avoided.

- When fat tissue becomes too thick, the circulation is affected. It is, therefore, important that the patient drinks water regularly and throughout the day – the *regularity is more important than the quantity consumed.* Warm water is better than cool, and it is surprising how quickly patients come to enjoy warm water.

- Finally, they should work daily at the area of the cellulite, massaging it with soft spiky toners and pummelling these areas so as to break the stagnation. Sitting cross-legged on the floor and moving sideways and forward and back in this position, causing friction on areas of cellulite ('bum walking'), for 15 minutes a day in the comfort of their home is an additional method to help improve circulation of blood flow.

7.11 SMALL BREASTS

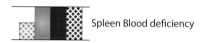

Spleen Blood deficiency

This is not a problem that patients generally come to an acupuncturist with – they would rather go to a surgeon. But, surprisingly, some patients who have come for other problems and have requested treatment for enlarging small breasts have experienced extremely good results.

7.11.1 Body acupuncture treatment

The Spleen is our organ of nutrition – it both receives and gives nutrition. Moreover, the breasts are on the Stomach meridian. So it seems logical that we should treat the Spleen for this problem. As we want to increase the size, we need to increase the Blood and yin. To achieve this, we can use the following points:

- Sp 3, Liv 13, Ren 17, Ren 12 and St 43 for Spleen and Stomach.

- Liv 1 and Liv 14 would tonify Liver yin as the Liver sends yin to the Stomach.

- P 6, UB 18 and UB 20 could help as general points.

These points could be alternated to use about 12 needles per session, treated twice weekly for 12 weeks. The results begin during the treatment, and continue well after. The same points can also be used to increase lactation. This treatment is not so successful if the patient is too thin.

7.11.2 What the patient can do at home

Patients should eat a 'damp-producing' diet. This dampness will settle where it is deficient, in this case in the breasts.

- They should drink full-fat milk twice daily and include some cheese and yoghurt in their diet.

- They should eat grains – white rice, millet, bread and pasta.

- They should eat more protein, especially chicken.

- Consuming a slow-cooked chicken soup with vegetables on a daily basis will help to increase the Spleen Blood.

7.12 LARGE AND HEAVY BREASTS

 Excess dampness in Spleen (and Liver) with or without Qi deficiency

This is caused by an excess of dampness in the Spleen, with or without Qi deficiency. It could also be part of Liver Blood stagnation. Women often complain of breast distension, pain and heaviness during the premenstrual period. This can be relieved by using points to sedate Spleen and Liver yin with one treatment – in fact, the patient feels well before the needles are even out. In the case of large breasts, we can apply needles to the same points for a longer time. During the menopause, women tend to put on weight, and often their breasts increase in size. These points are useful in both cases.

7.12.1 Body acupuncture treatment

- UB 18 and UB 20 – needle for 10 minutes, then dry cup for 10 minutes (the use of cupping on Back-Shu points helps to reduce dampness in the organ).

- Sp 9 (look for the tender point) and St 40.

- Liv 2 (sedation point), GB 37 (Luo-point, to sedate yin and tonify Qi).

- TW 5, UB 39 and lower sea point of the Triple Warmer (to improve circulation of dampness).

7.12.2 What the patient can do at home

- Avoid damp-producing foods.
- Drink water.
- Avoid coffee and alcohol.
- Be physically active and exercise regularly.

7.13 OBESITY

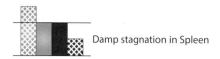

Damp stagnation in Spleen

This book would not be complete if I failed to mention obesity. Patients often ask to be treated to lose weight – and this is not at all easy to achieve. Nevertheless, there is some help we can give them.

An increase in weight often occurs in the later years of life – for example after childbirth, during menopause or with a change of lifestyle. The metabolic rate seems to slow down and enters into a vicious cycle of suppressing the Spleen Qi and the Qi of the Heart, Liver and Kidney. Treatment seems to work for short periods, but the weight and the old ways of eating and lifestyle seem to return.

The treatment I recommend is very successful, and worth a try.

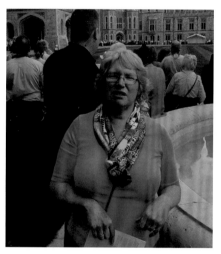

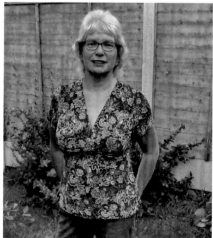

BEFORE   AFTER

I put the patients on a very low carbohydrate diet. They eat eggs, meat, fish, legumes, vegetables and fruit. They can also have hard cheese and nuts. I recommend three meals and two snacks daily. They should eat smaller quantities.

The patients seem to be able to follow the diet quite easily – and the weight loss is impressive. I have many patients who come for weight loss and they don't gain the weight back easily after this, so the treatment definitely seems to improve their metabolic rate.

7.13.1 Body acupuncture treatment

TO SEDATE SPLEEN DAMP AND TONIFY QI

- Sp 9, St 40, UB 20 and UB 21.

- Ren 12 with moxa only – given before the main meal time.

FOR TRANQUILLIZING AND AGAINST STRESS OR NERVOUSNESS

- Du 20, P 6.

- Liv 1 (this point is excellent for reducing craving for fatty and creamy foods).

- LI 4, TW 6 and St 25 (constipation points).

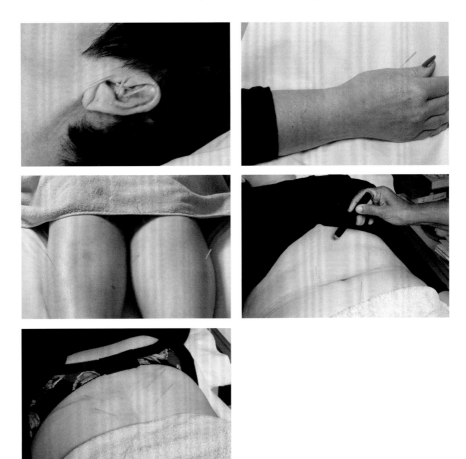

AGAINST SWEET CRAVINGS

- Sp 1 with moxa only (Ren 12 with moxa also helps).

Obese patients are often overweight in one area of the body. If they are overweight in the middle, the upper and lower warmers are often empty. In this case it is useful to tonify the yin and yang aspects of these warmers, in order to distribute the fullness evenly (Figures 7.13 and 7.14). It is also possible to break the stagnation in one body warmer, by working on the back:

- points to tonify upper warmer – Ren 14, Lu 1, UB 13, UB 15, P 6.

- points to tonify lower warmer – Ren 3, UB 23, UB 28, K 7 and UB 67.

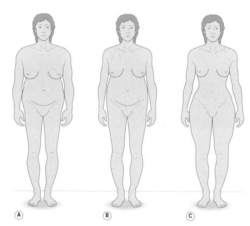

Figure 7.13 Three patterns of obesity. (A) Full upper warmer; (B) full middle warmer; (C) fullness of lower warmer

TREATMENT TO MOVE THE STAGNATION OF DAMPNESS AND FAT IN ONE WARMER

- The patient stands or lies on the abdomen for this treatment.

Tap with a plum-blossom hammer on a line 1 cm parallel to the back midline vertically downwards. The line should be tapped several times until a red skin reaction is obtained. The level of tapping is as follows:

- thorax – from the level of C6 to the level of T6.

- abdomen – from T7 to L2.

- lower abdomen – from L3 to S4.

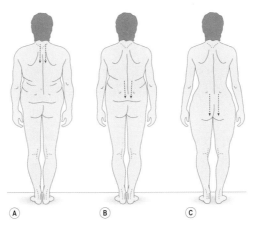

Figure 7.14 Lines for plum-blossom tapping to remove stagnation in the three patterns of obesity patterns of obesity

7.14 SUMMARY OF COSMETIC PROBLEMS AND ENERGY-BALANCING POINTS

TABLE 7.1 SUMMARY OF ENERGY-BALANCING POINTS

Problem	Imbalance		Treatment
Thin, wrinkly skin	Lung, Spleen and Kidney		Lu 1, Lu 9, Ren 17, Sp 3, K 10, drink more fluids and humidify rooms
Hanging, puffy skin	Spleen		UB 20, St 36, Sp 1, moxa
Swollen face	Spleen		Sp 9, St 40, UB 20, needle and cupping
Swollen eyelids	Excessive dampness in Spleen		Sp 9, St 40, UB 20

cont.

Problem	Imbalance		Treatment
	Stagnation of damp in Spleen		Sp 9, St 40, UB 20
	Spleen Blood and Qi deficiency		Liv 13, UB 20, GB 20, LI 4
Dark rings below eyes	Kidney yin deficiency		K 7 or K 10
	Kidney yang deficiency		UB 23, K 3, UB 67
Dull skin	Lung, Kidney		UB 13, Lu 10, LI 11, UB 23, K 3, UB 67
Dull, lifeless hair	Kidney yang deficiency		UB 13, Lu 10, LI 11, UB 23, K3, UB 67
	Lung Qi deficiency		
Dry hair with dandruff	Lung, Kidney		Lu 1, Lu 9, Ren 17, K 7, K 10, Ren 3, Sp 6
Cellulite	Damp stagnation in Spleen and affected meridian		UB 20, St 40. Gall Bladder: UB 19, GB 37. Urinary Bladder: UB 28, UB 58
Small breasts	Spleen (Liver) Blood deficiency		Sp 3, Liv 13, Ren 17, Ren 12, St 43, Liv 1, Liv 14
Large, heavy breasts	Excess dampness in Spleen and Liver		UB 18 and UB 20 needle and cupping, Sp 9, St 40, Liv 2, GB 37, TW 5, UB 39
Obesity	Damp stagnation in Spleen		Sp 9, St 40, UB 20, UB 21, P 6, Liv 1, Ren 12 and Sp 1 (both with moxa)

CHAPTER 8

NOTES FOR PATIENTS

The very first time a patient requests cosmetic therapy with acupuncture, I ask them what they are willing to do to achieve and maintain results. As cosmetic treatment costs over double the price of normal treatment, patients often ask how long the effect will last – and I always tell them that it depends on them. I find it is very good to instill this way of thinking in patients right from the beginning – so that they take responsibility for themselves. If they change their diet and their lives around their own needs, then they will improve tremendously under treatment.

However, there are some patients who resist changing anything at all but expect the treatment to change them and the effect to continue forever. I make an interesting comparison for them about the egg and the heat: 'If you want to get a chick out of an egg, you should apply heat; but you can apply all the heat you want to a stone, and it will not hatch into a chicken.'

We are the heat – and now it is in the patient's hands to decide if he or she wishes to be the egg or the stone. Every patient gets to hear this story, and must make their decision before treatment begins.

In the following passages, I have some advice for patients. You can make your own advice sheets or you can simply print this off and give it to every patient. It makes the treatment more personalized.

FOR PATIENTS WITH ACNE VULGARIS

- Avoid refined sugars and chocolates.
- Avoid full-fat milk products.
- Avoid fried foods.
- Cut down on refined carbohydrates and eat wholegrain foods.

- Those who are constipated should make sure their bowels move regularly – take two teaspoons of linseed with cereal or muesli every morning.

- Eat a pear a day, either raw or stewed, including the skin.

- Do some skipping or trampolining.

- Clean the skin thoroughly in the mornings and evenings, and apply a hot towel near the skin to steam the skin for 5 minutes. Then apply a light moisturizer. Do not pick at the pimples.

- Crab apple – a preparation of Bach flower remedies is a natural cleanser for bowels and skin. Take two drops in a sip of water three times daily.

FOR PATIENTS WITH WIND-HEAT NEURODERMATITIS

- Drink water throughout the day, at least a sip every 20 minutes.

- Humidify rooms with water containers, potted plants, a water spray or electric humidifiers. Do not worry what other people think, they will probably do it too!.

- Use an aqueous cream after washing or bathing to cover all the skin, in order to seal in the fluid. Use cream on the skin whenever you feel it is dry.

- If your skin is very dry and you are on a salt-free diet, it may be useful to include some sea salt in your diet.

- Avoid alcohol (no red wine at all), citrus fruit such as oranges and grapefruit, pickled foods, tomatoes and juices from cartons. Juices made at home are fine as long as they are fresh and not citrus.

- Practise yoga or other relaxation techniques. Make sure you go to bed by 11.00 p.m. at the latest.

- Avoid nylon and wool clothes. Whenever possible, use cotton next to the skin.

FOR PATIENTS WITH DAMP-HEAT TYPE ECZEMA

- Drink water regularly. Warm water is better than cool water.

- Avoid full-fat milk products and cheese.

- Avoid refined (white) carbohydrates – bread, rice, pasta – and eat wholegrain foods instead.

- Eat red meat no more than once a week.

- Do some physical exercise daily – even if it is only walking.

- Bathe in warm water containing two mugs of salt, once a week.

For patients with damp-cold type psoriasis

- Make a hot bath with 1 kg of sea salt and lie in it, topping up the hot water, for 20 minutes. Do this once a week.

Tips to improve dull hair and skin and general vitality

- Massage the roots of your hair with olive oil or coconut oil. Brush vigorously from the scalp to the tip several times. Wrap your head in a warm towel and keep warm for 20 minutes or leave oil on overnight. Wash off. Repeat once every week.

- Exercise regularly – walk or run 5 days a week for 30 minutes.

- Eat any type of fish, especially red fish (colour of flesh when raw).

- When cooking meat or poultry, use the bones and legs to make stock and chew on the bone when possible. Eat the deep-fried or pressure-cooked bones of small fish; these are very good nutrition for the Kidney yang.

- Bring more romance into your life and enjoy regular sex.

- Hang your head below bed level for 10 minutes every day – this brings blood flow to the head and face, increasing the shine of skin and hair.

What to do to counter swollen, puffy eyelids

- Dissolve two tablespoons of sea salt in a cup of water; thinly slice a cucumber and soak the slices in this water. Store in the refrigerator. Lie down and place the cucumber slices on the eyelids for 10 minutes (keep eyes shut) before washing off. Try not to get any salt water in the eyes as it will sting.

- Avoid eating after 6.00 p.m. If hungry, eat a light minestrone soup.

How to prevent and treat wrinkles at home

- Use an egg face pack, prepared as follows. Beat a whole egg in a bowl. Using a brush, paint your face and neck with the egg. Repeat after 10 minutes. Wait until it dries well – do not make facial expressions during this time. Wash off 20 minutes after the second application. Use a light moisturizer afterwards, as the egg is quite drying.

- Mung bean face pack. Soak green mung beans (broken) overnight in water. Grind them in a wet grinder or processor the next morning. Spread as a thick paste on your face and neck (this is also very good for the hair, but is difficult to remove before washing). After 30 minutes, remove the paste. Wash face and moisturize.

These two packs are nourishing for the skin and can be applied once weekly. The mung paste mask will also help to remove facial hair. However, both face masks are quite drying and the skin needs to be moisturized afterwards.

To treat thin and wrinkly skin

- Do not smoke.

- Consume a quarter-litre tub of buttermilk per day.

- Drink water throughout the day.

- Eat watery fruits and vegetables such as melon, grapes and cucumber.

- Eat foods pre-soaked or cooked in water (as opposed to smoked and baked) – they have more water energy.

- Eat stews and slow-cooked foods – they increase dampness.

- Humidify rooms with a water container, water spray, potted plants or humidifier.

- Eat a small bowl of white rice daily.

- Apply a rich cream after bathing in order to help the skin retain water.

- Avoid coffee, alcohol and direct sun exposure.

WHAT TO DO TO COUNTER A SWOLLEN FACE, OBESITY OR CELLULITE

- Avoid full-fat milk and dairy products.

- Avoid refined carbohydrates and sugars.

- Avoid raw and cold foods.

- Drink warm water.

- Avoid thick sauces and soups – more watery sauces and soups are better.

- Have a hearty breakfast, moderate lunch and a light evening meal before 6.00 p.m. A watery soup made from onions, leeks, spinach, celery, tomato, mushroom and cabbage with a small amount of meat or fish for flavour is a good evening meal. Two or three small bowls of this soup can be eaten in the evening if the patient is particularly hungry.

- Patients who feel they are missing out on family time can use the evenings to take a walk, go for a swim or play a game with their family instead of sitting at the table. If the family's main meal is in the evening, set aside your portion and store it in the fridge for lunch the following day.

- Regular exercise – 30 minutes five times a week – is essential. The exercise should increase the heart rate – a brisk walk, run or swim would be ideal. Sport, aerobic exercise and martial arts are especially good; older patients could do toning and stretching, yoga, Tai Ji or Qi Gong and some cardiovascular exercise.

- For patients who suffer from heartburn, a teaspoon of honey mixed in warm water taken 20 minutes before a meal is beneficial. For patients who feel heavy and lethargic after a meal, the same honey drink can be consumed after a meal to aid digestion.

WHAT CAN BE DONE TO COUNTER HYPERPIGMENTATION

- Avoid exposure to the sun.

- Boil milk until a skin forms. Skim off the skin and store it in a saucer in the fridge. Apply it to the dark skin – if too dry, moisten with some milk. Wash off after 10 minutes.

CHAPTER 9

FIVE ELEMENTS AND FACIAL TYPES
Problems and Corrections

Since I practice Five Element acupuncture, this book would not be complete without mention of some of the typical cosmetic problems related to the particular element associated with a facial type.

9.1 FACIAL TYPES

9.1.1 Fire element

Common characteristics

- These patients tend to have a reddish complexion (or an absence of colour) in their faces).

    - A red face (together with other characteristics described here) generally suggests Heart yang excess.

    - When the face is pale but with red areas on the cheeks and neck, this may indicate Heart yin deficiency with a tendency to rising yang.

    - An absence of red colour on the face (again, with the other characteristics described here), could mean Heart Blood deficiency.

- They tend to have a smallish head, pointed chin and less hair (if Heart yin is deficient), or curly hair (if Heart yang is deficient).

- They are quick, active and energetic.

- They are analytical and inquisitive.

- In all deficienciency states, they will tend to have small extremities.

Depending on whether they are red faced, pale faced or pale with red areas, they will need to be treated accordingly.

- Red face – often feet are colder.

  - Treat with Sp 6 descending technique, K 4, Ren 3 and SI 8 sedation.

- Pale face – Blood deficiency or Heart yang deficiency.

  - Blood deficiency – Ren 14, UB15, UB 17, Sp 10, GB 39

  - Heart yang deficiency – UB 15, H 3, SI 3.

- Red areas – Heart yin deficiency, yang rising.

  - Treat with H 5, Ren 14, K 7.

- They suffer with insomnia and are easily tired.

  - Treat with Du 20, Ex 6, An Mian 1, UB 62.

- They can have performance anxiety, which they show by wringing their hands and quick darting of eyes – Heart yin deficiency.

  - Treat with H 9, Ren 14, Du 20 and P 6.

- They smile or laugh easily – tending to get lines around the eyes. They think a lot (not worry) causing lines between the brows. They are always in a rush, doing things at the last minute.

TREATMENT

Lines between brows caused by concentration can be treated using the following methods:

- Gua Sha massage
- Individual wrinkle treatment
- By increasing their awareness of this body language
- Encourage them to think with their eyes closed, and placing their hands by their sides
- Mental relaxation exercises daily in the evening before bed
- Foot massage or warm foot bath to descend the heat and energy.

9.1.2 Earth element

Common characteristics

- They have a yellowish complexion (pale and yellow in Spleen Blood and Qi deficiency).

- They tend to have rather a big head with a round face (this is possible even if the person is not obese).

- There is a tendency towards large abdomen and limbs with well-built muscles.

- They have a heavy walk with large thighs and calves.

- They move little, preferring to sit.

- They are worriers, with lines across the forehead and around the eyes, and a deep naso-labial groove.

- Excessive dampness causes them to have heavy jowls.

- Their oral body language leads to lines around the lips.

- They can have large and heavy breasts (excessive damp) or small breasts (Spleen Blood deficiency).

TREATMENT

- Strengthen the sides of the face and the back of neck with needles (lifting procedure)
- Treat the naso-labial groove with needles in the same way as for a wrinkle
- Treat the jowls and heavy cheeks with cupping before Gua Sha massage
- Needle the Back-shu points, Moxa the Du meridian, and back massage to strengthen the back and straighten and improve the posture (because the patient tends to hunch forward)
- Treat lip lines with Gua Sha and lip contour with needles
- Points UB 20, Sp 9 and St 40 to tonify Spleen Qi
- Advise patients to eat lightly in the evenings
- Milk products only in moderation after 3.00 p.m.
- They should use oil only as a marinade, not to cook with
- They should avoid refined carbohydrates and sweets
- They should take regular and moderate exercise.

9.1.3 Metal element

Common characteristics

- They tend to be pale faced (they may have red blotchy areas on face and neck) – Lu yin deficiency.

- They are square faced, with a small face, upper body and hands.

- They have a tendency towards dry skin (in the case of Lung yin deficiency) or oily skin (shows dampness in Lung) in the upper body. The skin of the lower body may be different.

- They have a nasal body language.

- They may suffer with chronic sinusitis, post-nasal drip and oedema around the sinus area – stagnation of dampness – this is not necessarily due to excessive dampness (though it could be if the patient consumes excessive dairy or refined carbohydratess or sweets), and could also be because the mucus is too thick (yin deficiency).

- They can be quite wrinkly (like smokers), making them look older than their age – Lung yin deficiency. If the skin is dry and thin, this could be additionally Lung Blood deficiency.

- They can also suffer from high or low pigmentation problems, especially in the face or upper body.

  o Hyperpigmentation shows that the yang is high. This may be due to exposure or because the yin is low.

  o Depigmentation is a sign of low yang and Qi in the Lung.

- They may have itchy eyes and itchy areas around the nose – usually a cause of dark rings around the eyes. This is a result of wind-heat attacking the skin as in allergies. Though the eye is related to the Liver, the sclera and conjunctiva of the eye (i.e. the skin of the eye) are governed by the Lung. Irritation of the eye that occurs during the allergy season is therefore seen as a wind-heat symptom of the Lung.

TREATMENT

- To tonify Lung yin use points Lu 1, Lu 7 (needle obliquely towards the wrist), K 10, Sp 3 and Ren 17 upward needling
- Treat with Gua Sha once weekly, treat stubborn wrinkles with needles
- Humidify rooms and patient should drink water regularly
- Consume a quarter of a litre of buttermilk (or lassi) each morning
- Patients should learn to empty their sinuses after steam inhalation
- Nasal allergies should be treated, add also Sp 10, GB 20
- Patients should remove allergens from living spaces.

9.1.4 Water element

Common characteristics

- They have either a large lower body (Kidney yang deficiency) or a narrower lower body (Kidney yin deficiency).

- They have a long spine.

- Their skin may appear wrinkled (yin deficiency) or look filled and shiny (yang deficiency with yin stagnation).

- They tend to have dark rings below their eyes, dark colour on their cheeks or a dark coating on the tongue – this can mean that either Kidney yin or yang or both aspects are deficient.

- They can either have a defined jaw with a protruding chin (yang-dominant Kidney state); or they have a loose chin contour, philtrum and floppy neck.

- Acne in the area around the mouth before periods is a sign of damp-heat in Ming-men (reproductive) Kidneys.

- Their skin looks uneven, and their body shakes (like waves) when walking.

TREATMENT

- Kidney yin deficiency manifests as a smaller lower body with rising heat, restlessness in the Heart and hot flushes
  - Treat with K 4 alternating with K 7, Ren 3, Ren 24, Lu 7, UB 40, Sp 6
- Kidney yang deficiency manifests as a looser and larger lower part of face and body
  - Treat with K 3, UB 67, UB 23 (needle and cupping), UB 28, St 36
  - Use para-vertebral tapping with a plum-blossom hammer at L2–S4 to improve firmness
  - Cup (six large cups) at L2–S4 to counter oedema
  - Use lifting needles on the parietal and occipital areas of the head and neck in order to firm the lower part of the face and neck.

9.1.5 Wood element

Common characteristics

- The wood type could have either a pale face, which indicates Blood deficiency, or a red face and red eyes, which is a sign of Liver yang excess.

- They are not physical workers but are intellectuals, and as such tend to have a slim body with a small head, hands and feet.

- They have a tendency towards nervousness, and sometimes tics or tremors.

- They have an eye-related body language – squinting, glaring or irritation of the eyes. These are mostly wind symptoms, whereas glaring is more of a Liver yang excess symptom.

- They are susceptible to neck tension and tension headaches on the side or the occipital region of the head.

- Physical strain may cause tendon problems.

- Tension may also cause wind symptoms such as wandering pains, muscle colic and sudden vomiting or breathing problems.

- Excessive tension can lead to high Blood pressure and flaccid muscle tension may result in low Blood pressure.

TREATMENT

- Pale face – Liver Blood deficiency
  - Tonify the Blood: Ren 14, UB 15, UB 17, Gb 39, Sp 10
- Red face – Liver yang excess, yin deficiency
  - Tonify the yin, sedate the yang: Liv 5, GB 40 sedation, Lu 7, Sp 6
- Nervousness, tics or tremor
  - Tonify the Liver yin: Liv 5, K 7, Lu 1, Du 20
  - Electrical stimulation with continuous frequency on the muscle to counter tics
- Tension
  - Same as above with local points on the tense area
- Wind symptoms
  - Wind elimination tonification or sedation accordingly (pages 103–105)
- Squinting of eyes
  - Ex 2, UB 2, Gb 37
- Sunken eyes – Liver Blood deficiency
  - Add Blood deficiency points with Liv 1, Lu 1, K 7.

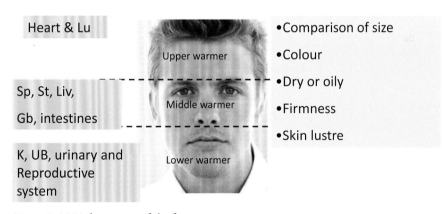

Heart & Lu

Sp, St, Liv, Gb, intestines

K, UB, urinary and Reproductive system

Upper warmer

Middle warmer

Lower warmer

- Comparison of size
- Colour
- Dry or oily
- Firmness
- Skin lustre

Figure 9.1 Triple warmer of the face

9.2 WHAT WE CAN DO WITH THE TRIPLE WARMER?

When treating the symmetry of our face, the Triple Warmer is very useful and important. We look at the Triple Warmer as a whole, but also as three separate parts, just as our body has three parts – the upper body, middle body and lower body. The appearance of our tongue also shows the state of the Blood, yin, yang and energy states in the three areas.

The energy state in the upper, middle and lower body can be determined by reading the pulse:

- The *distal pulses* show the upper body energies – Heart and Lung.

- The *middle position* shows the middle body energies – Liver and Spleen.

- At the *proximal pulse position* we can palpate the lower body energies – both the water aspect and the reproductive aspect of the Kidneys.

On the face:

- The upper warmer is reflected in the forehead area – above the brows, including the temples; the area extends to the scalp in the frontal region of the head.

- The middle warmer is represented by the middle of the face, from below the eyebrows to just below the nose (Figure 9.1).

- The lower warmer is represented by the area from above the lips to the end of the chin; the area extends to the front of the neck.

- The sensory organs in any area here are considered as part of the main organs – eyes to the Liver and lips to the Spleen and so on.

When working with the symmetry of the areas of the Triple Warmer, we should look at:

- Size.

- Colour.

- Firmness.

- Dry or oily.

- Skin lustre.

9.2.1 Comparison of size and tension

- *Larger area* may mean:

  ○ Fullness (excess yin or dampness).

- ○ Looseness or flaccidity (Qi deficiency).

Example:

- Swollen eyelids – caused by excessive dampness in the Spleen.

    - ○ Treat with Sp 9 with or without sedation technique.

    - ○ Use cupping locally; salt cucumber for 15 minutes to reduce the oedema.

- Sagging or drooping eyelids – Spleen and Stomach Qi deficiency.

    - ○ Treat with UB 20/21, Sp 1, St 40.

    - ○ Use plum-blossom tapping or Gua Sha locally to lift.

    - ○ Give needles to lift the brow.

- *Smaller area* could be:

    - ○ Emptiness (Blood deficiency).

    - ○ High tension (yin deficiency).

Example:

- Small forehead: St/LI yin deficiency.

    - ○ Tonify yin with Ren 12, St 43, P 6 for Stomach.

    - ○ Tonify yin with St 25, LI 5 and Lu 8 for Large Intestine.

- High tension around eyes – Liver yin deficiency.

    - ○ Tonify Liver yin with Liv 1 or 14, Lu 7, K 7.

9.2.2 Dry or oily

- Treat greasiness or damp acne as dampness with:

    - ○ Back-shu points of organs.

    - ○ Luo-connecting points of yang organs.

    - ○ Local cupping and local needling.

- Treat dryness, fine wrinkles with:

    - ○ Local Gua Sha.

- Tonify yin of relevant organs with Front-mu points, own element points in yin organs and grandmother points of yang organs.

Example:

- Dry, flaky itchy scalp with little red pimples on forehead and near hairline – Lung yin deficiency with wind-heat.

  - Lu 1, 8, Ren 17, St 25, LI 5, K 10.

  - Use warm oil on scalp and leave for 20 minutes or overnight before washing.

  - Lastly, rinse with vinegar water (add a cup of vinegar to a large bowl of warm water).

- Oily skin with large pustules around the jawline – damp-heat in Kidneys.

  - UB 23/28, UB 58, St 40, Ren 3, Sp 6, LI 4.

  - Treat with many superficial local needles.

9.2.3 Colour and lustre

- Redness and wind-heat acne in an area – yin deficiency in organs in area, wind-heat.

  - Tonify yin of organs as before.

  - Wind elimination sedation on GB 20 (see page 105 for technique).

- 'Unclean' complexion in area – Qi deficiency of the organs.

  - Local steaming.

  - Tonify Qi of organ using Back-shu points and Luo point of yang organ.

- Mixed skin on face – Spleen Qi deficiency.

  - UB 20, St 36, Sp 1.

CHAPTER 10

A PERSONAL NOTE

Dear reader, in this book I have shared my experiences with you. Most of these have been good. However, over the years I have learned not to do certain things. I would like to share these with you as well.

Most of the patients I take on for cosmetic acupuncture therapy are already my acupuncture patients. I have previously known them, having treated them for other problems, and we are comfortable with each other. When they hear about my work with cosmetic problems, they express curiosity and we talk about it. Eventually, they decide to try it. Most of them will continue to have treatment once every 2 or 3 months after an initial set of six to eight sessions.

I rarely treat patients who are not on my patient list although, occasionally, a relative of an existing patient may come along with them for cosmetic therapy.

Patients requesting cosmetic acupuncture are usually women aged 40–56 years. They are usually working women, financially independent, open to alternative medicine and take pride in being able to take care of themselves and their families. They are aware of the side-effects of medication, and will not rush to take painkillers, hormones or antidepressants at the first sign of a problem. They will read up on the problems they have, and are well informed.

I really enjoy working with this client group. I learn as much from them as they do from me. They inform me about current therapies and clinics, and this helps me to keep up to date with what I offer my patients. They report overreactions to my treatment immediately, and trust me enough to return to me so that I can correct my mistakes. I am truly grateful to these patients of mine, without whom I would have nothing to write about in this book today.

There have also been difficult patients, pathologically demanding ones, who I have regretted taking on as cosmetic patients. There are some patients who come in expecting the moon, or are very enthusiastic at the beginning but lose interest and fail to attend appointments as time goes on.

The following are some decisions I have made over the course of time:

- Do not accept cosmetic patients 1 or 2 weeks before a special occasion (such as a wedding or holiday) unless they have already had at least three or four sessions.

- For an eight-session course of expensive therapies such as face lifting or laser with hyaluronic acid, the patient is asked to pay 50 per cent of the total cost in advance. Thereafter, they need pay only 50 per cent of the cost of the individual treatments. I believe that this payment schedule increases patients' commitment and, having already paid half the fee, they do not find it difficult to pay the remainder.

- Choose patients who are easy or not too difficult to work with. Do not accept very difficult cases for cosmetic acupuncture.

- Do not agree to treat wrinkles in smokers.

- I give patients body acupuncture as the first part of each treatment, and the cosmetic procedure follows this. Patients have to follow a list of dos and don'ts at home. Do not compromise on this.

- Do not treat patients for cosmetic reasons if they are ill (e.g. with flu, the common cold or a cough) on that day.

- Allow 1½ hours for each appointment, even though you may need only 1 hour. The patient could bleed or faint, and it is necessary to leave time to deal with this. Patients should not feel rushed. I normally see several patients in different rooms, but I keep one room available in the event of extra time being required.

- Never promise a patient the moon. I never tell them I can cure – only that I will try my best and that I have treated this problem successfully before, but each patient is unique. If improvement is going to be achieved, it will be seen within the first few sessions, in which case the treatment can continue. If no benefit is apparent after five sessions then I recommend stopping treatment, to which patients usually agree.

- Do not capitalize on patients' anxiety and agree to treat too many conditions at the same time, or to give treatments too often. Some patients request treatment for five different ailments and cosmetic acupuncture at the same time. Although it is possible to treat more than one problem at the same time, treating too many conditions concurrently means that no treatment is successful. Advise patients that treatment of symptoms should be prioritized and that you will not compromise on this.

- Charge patients for missed appointments. Even if you know them well, charge at least a nominal fee. You have put aside an hour and a half for them, and this time is now wasted.

- Most of your cosmetic patients will continue to come to you about four to six times a year. Balance their energy and keep them young and you will get their spouses, children, grandchildren and more as your patients for many years to come.

This book deals with theory and practice, needling and other techniques to treat dermatology and cosmetic problems. Techniques – however sophisticated – are not enough in clinical practice. The practitioner's approach, the client–practitioner relationship and, above all, the attitude of the practitioner towards his or her work and patients are all crucial for effective clinical work. While most of the knowledge and skills involved in cosmetic acupuncture can be taught, these aspects of practice referred to above are founded on the practitioner's basic values and professionalism.

The ethical principle of beneficence obliges therapists to treat their clients in a way that produces maximum benefit. Clients request cosmetic treatments for a variety of reasons, ranging from wanting to look better to a self-centred obsession with good looks. Some demanding clients may evoke strong emotional reactions in the therapist. However, it is not for therapists to judge their clients – rather they should respect the clients' wishes, feelings and requests. This is not always easy, especially for the beginners in cosmetic acupuncture. The therapist needs to learn the difference between the feelings the client brings into the session and the strong emotional reactions these produce in the therapist.

The best way to overcome the above pitfalls and traps is to ask yourself: am I adhering to the basic ethical principles and values – honesty, integrity, respect for clients – that underpin my practice? Am I being 100 per cent professional in my approach?

There are a number of challenges to preserving our professionalism in our practice and it is easy to fall into traps if one is not consciously aware of them. These include the following:

- Commercialization: charging a fee for each item of service can tempt therapists to continue treatment longer than is necessary. The body acupuncture session and cosmetic needling is part of the same treatment, and cannot be billed separately.

- Consumerism: the client should not be allowed to pressurize the therapist into undertaking therapies that will not be effective.

- Industrialization: the temptation to operate like an 'assembly line', to maximize the number of patients seen, can lead to loss of control over holistic care.

While the above challenges are common to all clinical practices, they are more acute and demanding in cosmetic acupuncture, and the temptation to violate basic ethical principles is ever-present. We should always bear in mind that we are primarily acupuncture practitioners who heal patients. We deliver cosmetic therapies in the process of offering acupuncture to balance the body energies. A great deal of skill and expertise underlie our cosmetic therapies and we must always be aware of the professional obligations and demands that are placed upon us as practitioners.

I have had many enjoyable years working in cosmetic acupuncture, and I wish you as much fun and joy and great achievements from reading this book and implementing the ideas outlined here.

GLOSSARY

ACNE

A disorder of sebaceous glands and hair follicles of the skin, characterized by papules and pustules.

ACUPUNCTURE

A form of Chinese treatment using needles.

ACUPUNCTURE ANALGESIA

Pain relief using acupuncture.

ALOPECIA

Loss of head hair, baldness.

ALOPECIA AREATA

Hair loss in sharply defined areas.

ANAL FISSURE

Slit in the mucous membrane of the anus.

BACK-SHU POINTS

Two points at either side of the vertebral prominence which govern the function of different organs. The Back-Shu points are also called positive reaction points, meaning that these points become tender or develop tension or nodes when organs in the area suffer dysfunction. Needling these points cures the dysfunction and diminishes the positive reaction. As these points are on the back and therefore the yang surface of the body, they influence the yang aspect or the function of the organs.

BLOOD

Red blood, nutrition, enables healing, circulates warmth.

BOTOX

A trade name for a preparation of botulinum toxin. Botulinum toxin is a neurotoxin protein produced by the bacterium Clostridium botulinum. Minute doses of this are used to treat painful muscle spasms, and to smooth facial wrinkles.

CELLULITE

A fatty deposit causing a dimpled appearance, usually in the skin of the lower limbs, abdomen and pelvis region.

CIRRHOSIS

A chronic disease of the liver characterized by replacement of normal tissue with fibrous tissue and loss of functional liver cells.

CYANOSIS

A bluish discoloration of the skin and mucous membrane resulting from inadequate oxygenation of the Blood.

DERMATOLOGY

The medical specialty concerned with the diagnosis and treatment of skin diseases.

DISPERSION

Moving from the interior towards the exterior.

DIURESIS

Increasing the excretion of urine.

DU MERIDIAN

The Du meridian is an extra meridian that is also called the Governor Vessel. It flows along the back midline of the body, and is considered to be the most yang meridian of the body. Tonifying the Du meridian can increase the general yang energy of the body. The Du and Ren meridians are considered to be extra meridians, and do not belong to any particular organ. They are coupled with each other.

EARTH

Element represented by the Spleen and Stomach organs, which receive, digest, absorb and distribute nutrition from food and drink to all the body.

ECZEMA

General term for any inflammation of skin (dermatitis), characterized by redness and itching, with or without discharge or scales.

ENDOGENOUS

From within; without cause from the exterior.

EPISTAXIS

A nose bleed.

ERYTHEMA

Red patches, usually raised above skin surface, sometimes itchy or painful.

FIRE

Heat. The element is represented by two pairs of organs – the Heart and the Small Intestine and the Pericardium and the Triple Warmer.

DISPERSING FIRE NEEDLE TECHNIQUE

Eliminates heat from a meridian/organ.

FRONT-MU POINT

Also called the alarm-point, where pain appears when organs are diseased. Needling this point can alleviate the pain and correct the dysfunction.

FUNCTIONAL ENERGY

Energy used in creating the function of a tissue or organ.

FURUNCULOSIS

The simultaneous occurrence of a number of furuncles (boils).

GUA SHA METHOD

A therapy using a flat instrument to scrape the skin to bring the pathogenic energy from the exterior tissues to the surface.

HEAT

Feeling of heat, inflammation, restlessness, redness.

HYPERHIDROSIS

Excessive sweating.

HYPERMENORRHOEA (MENORRHAGIA)

Excessive menstrual bleeding.

HYPERPIGMENTATION

Excess pigmentation (darker colouring) of the skin or mucous membrane.

HYPODERMIC

Applied or administered beneath the skin.

IDIOPATHIC ITCHING

Itching for which no particular cause has been found.

LUO-CONNECTING POINT

A point of a meridian that connects to the coupled meridian. It is considered to be a single point that can balance two meridians, especially when there is an excess in one and a deficiency in the other. I use the Luo-connecting point of the yin meridian if the yin is deficient and the yang is in excess; and the Luo-connecting point of the yang meridian if the yang is deficient and the yin is in excess.

MALAR FLUSH

Redness of the cheeks.

METABOLISM

The processes involved in the transformation of nutrition to energy.

METAL

One of the five elements – metal represents the organs Lung and Large Intestine, and their physiological and pathological states in the body.

MOXA

Leaves of the mugwort (Artemesia vulgaris) dried and made into wool cigars to use directly over the skin or small caps to burn over needles.

MOXIBUSTION

Burning of moxa to warm the skin, a needle, an area or a meridian. Treatment is used in symptoms that worsen with exterior cold.

MUCOUS MEMBRANES

A membrane lining of most body cavities.

NEURODERMATITIS

Eczema of an unexplained origin. The term 'neuro' implies that the itching is of psychogenic origin. Dermatitis (inflammation of skin) in which localized areas (especially neck areas) itch persistently.

NUTRITION

Giving nourishment, endurance of function, ability to heal when injured or ill.

OEDEMA

Swelling, produced by excessive accumulation of watery fluid in tissue.

OWN-ELEMENT POINT

Each meridian has five element points (fire point, earth point, metal point, water point and wood point). One of these points will belong to the own element as the meridian (organ). This is called its own-element point (e.g. Lu 8 is the metal point of the Lung and St 36 is the earth point of the Stomach).

PATHOGENIC

Disease causing.

PLUM-BLOSSOM HAMMER

Short and light hammer with many short needles.

PLUM-BLOSSOM NEEDLE TAPPING

Tapping the skin lightly to cause a red skin reaction (increase the yang) or heavily to cause bleeding (to release heat).

PSORIASIS

Chronic skin disease characterized by dry, red patches covered with silvery white scales; occurs especially on the scalp, ears and skin covering bony prominences.

QI

Energy flow in meridians.

REN MERIDIAN

The Ren meridian is an extra meridian that flows on the front midline of the body. It is considered to be the most yin meridian of the body and can be used for tonifying the general yin of the body. There are many Front-mu points of the organs on the Ren meridian, which are used to influence the yin quality of 'cooling and calming' the organ.

SEBACEOUS SECRETION

Secretions from the sebaceous glands in the skin.

SEBORRHOEA

Excessive secretion of sebum resulting in an oily coating or crusts on the skin.

SEDATION

Dispersing or reducing energy with acupuncture.

SUBCUTANEOUS

Beneath the skin.

TACHYARRHYTHMIA

Fast and irregular heartbeat.

TACHYCARDIA

Fast heart rate.

TONIFICATION

Increasing and improving energy.

TRIPLE WARMER

The interior of the body where all internal organs are present. This is divided into three virtual warm spaces: the upper warmer is above the diaphragm (Heart and Lung); the middle warmer is in the centre (Liver, Gall Bladder, Spleen, Stomach, and Small and Large Intestines); the lower warmer is in the pelvis (Kidney and Urinary Bladder).

URTICARIA

An itchy skin eruption characterized by red, raised weals with well-defined margins; usually caused by allergy.

VITILIGO

A skin disease characterized by patches of depigmented skin (without colour).

WATER

One of the five elements, represented by the organs Kidney and Urinary Bladder, which store water and irrigate the body.

WIND

Can be climatic or generated by the Liver in the interior; it is important for moving blood, energy and fluid in the body and to remove stagnation. Excessive wind may cause irritating and wandering symptoms.

WOOD

One of the five elements, represented by the Liver and Gall Bladder, which help control muscles and tendons – their function, flexibility and strength.

YANG

Co-exists with yin. Represents heat, activity, change, upward and outward movement, daytime and power.

YIN

Co-exists with yang. Represents cold, passivity and rest, stability, downward and inward movement, night-time and nutrition and endurance.

ZANG FU

The 12 main internal organs of the body, also called solid and hollow organs.

INDEX

Sub-headings in *italics* indicate tables.